THE ELEPHANT'S ROPE
AND
THE UNTETHERED SPIRIT

*A Remarkable, True Story
of Healing and Hope*

Lynne Picard

Robert D. Reed Publishers
San Francisco

Robert D. Reed Publishers
750 LaPlaya, Suite 647
San Francisco, CA 94121
Phone: 650-994-6570 • Fax: -6579
E-mail: 4bobreed@msn.com
http://www.rdrpublishers.com

Typesetter: Barbara Kruger
Cover design: Irene Taylor, it grafx

ISBN 1-885003-25-0

Library of Congress Catalog Card Number 99-066909

Manufactured, typeset and printed in the United States of America

DEDICATION

For My Family and Friends, Healers, Angels and Doctors,
For Lugard Road and The Lake in the Sky,
For Lotte at my feet,
And, of course, for Nana then and now.

ACKNOWLEDGEMENTS

At a dinner party several years ago I was encouraged by an old friend in the publishing world to put my experiences, some of which she had previously heard about, on paper. In fact, in the form of a literary sketchbook, I had already begun. When the rudimentary collection of pages was ready, Connie Roosevelt continued her support and agreed to make the first pass at editing my fledgling manuscript, starting me off in the very best direction. For this I am extremely grateful.

More than a year later, Valerie Andrews came along at the right moment and fine-tuned the work that had been done in the interim, professionally and with enthusiastic encouragement. Again I am extremely grateful.

Special thanks to Suzanne McConnell, a fine writer, friend and instructor at Hunter College, who read the first galleys and gave fresh insights, providing better, more precise words to phrases which had become too familiar to be improved upon from within, and saved me from many red pencil errors.

And finally I met Colin Ingram, Senior Editor for Monterey Pacific Publishers, who writes beautifully, does a masterful job, and is a pleasure to work with. Thank you for believing in me.

And to Robert Reed, for his patience, support, and expertise.

On a journey seeking wellness and illumination like this one, the quality and length of my trip has been enhanced by fine healers and teachers who have become special friends. With the exception of one, these friends had not come into my life before 1991 when this written story ends; but they are all a blessed part of it, and a part of my being here. I am thankful not only for the support and friendship they have given, but for the quality of information bestowed and exchanged. I am so glad for the laughter and pleasure of our collaborations, the miracles shared.

Connie Arismende in Lemmon Valley, Nevada; Susan Bryant and Sandy Burns at Earth Elements in Flagstaff, Arizona; Dorothy Dunn in San Clemente, California; Dr. Willard Fuller in Fairburn, Georgia; Father Joshua in Sedona, Arizona; Margarette French in Peng Chau, Hong Kong; David Fuess, in Pacific Grove, California; Beth Gray in Woodside, California; Anneliese Hagemann in Wautoma, Wisconsin; Tricia Korte in Monterey, California; Jason Mixter in San Francisco, California; Doug Mitchell in Grass Valley, California; Sara Niccolls in Ross, California; Dr. Dickey Nyeronsha in Berkeley, California; Angela Rennilson in Monterey, California; and Greg Schelkun, in San Rafael, California.

And to my wonderful friends who have encouraged and buttressed the desire to do justice to my little story, even when it meant disappearing for hours, or not answering telephone calls for days and, in some time zones, weeks: you are all treasures, adding bubbles and joy and unbelieveable varieties of wisdom. I am so glad and grateful to have you in my life:

Alice Bahrenburg, Joanne Bjork, Tink Davis, Suzette James, Elizabeth Jowett, Cindy Kantner, Sydney Kapchan, Susie McBaine, (cover artist extraordinaire), Smudge McVickar, Beth Terrell, Cia and SteveTownsend, Virginia Veach, and the many others who have so enriched and inspired my life without knowing what I was up to.

And to my dear family, all of whom I love so much. Geoff, Lex and Tim, Peter, and Coco, Lotte, Victoria and Leo, thank you for supporting me, especially in the times when you weren't quite sure where I was going. And to my mother and father, to Cindy and Bob, Kirsten and Dan, Allison, Bauma, Shirley, Shirley and Bill, I love you all and am so grateful to have such a warm, loving family. You are all in my heart.

HOPE

As I ate breakfast one morning, I overheard two oncologists conversing. One complained bitterly: "You know, Bob, I just don't understand it. We used the same drugs, the same dosage, the same schedule and the same entry criteria. Yet I got a 22 percent response rate and you got a 74 percent. That's unheard of for metastatic cancer. How do you do it?"

His colleague replied, "We're both using Etoposide, Platinum, Oncovin and Hydroxyurea. You call yours EPOH. I tell my patients I'm giving them HOPE. As dismal as the statistics are, I emphasize that we have a chance."

—William M. Buchholz, M.D.

Reprinted with permission of the author

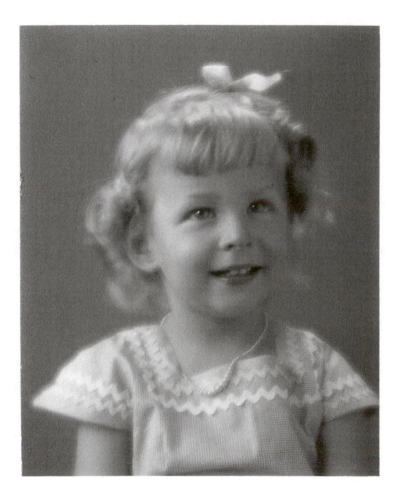

Introduction

When we returned to India for a visit several years ago, I became acquainted with a beautiful elephant and her master. They were both elegantly dressed, selling bumpy rides up to and down from the old Amber Palace in Jaipur. The elephant was well cared for, with vividly colored designs chalked onto her body from ear to ear, and wherever else the large saddle didn't cover. Her master wore a white khadi-cloth dhoti with a brilliantly colored hot pink turban and a grand old graying handlebar moustache, of which he was understandably proud. He was a small, wiry man. He sat upon the elephant's head and carried a whip, which he waved in the air but never used on the animal.

While resting between work periods, it was puzzling to notice that the elephant seemed to be kept from roaming by a very thin rope, tied around one of her back legs and then to a heavy piece of scruffy undergrowth. The master routinely squatted down and smoked with his friends nearly 50 yards away, a distance which, it seemed, would have given him very little influence over the elephant's mobility. The power of the rope was definitely perplexing. With a very slight pull this large animal could surely have escaped, or at least chosen to wander where she pleased. Perhaps she simply didn't want to. I wondered about it.

With help from an English-speaking guide it was easy to find out. In Hindi he proposed my question to the proud old boy in the hot pink turban.

"Wouldn't your elephant run off if she wanted to?"

Characteristically twisting his head from side to side in the manner of Indians, he replied, "Yes, Sa'hib. Of course, Sa'hib."

"Then why doesn't she? The rope is small. She could easily break it."

"Yes, Sa'hib. But when she was a baby, a chain was put around her leg and then around a tree. She tried to break it but she couldn't. After a while she didn't try. I put the thin rope on her now because she doesn't

1

know that she could break it. Her idea about it is from when she was small."

It was an exotically odd, somehow charming story. I tucked it into my rich bag of experiences.

Years later, while striving to heal my life and body from cancer, the story came back quite unexpectedly one day as a metaphor. Without knowing it, I, too, had been bound by an assortment of emotional, intellectual, and psychological ropes – chains which had powerfully transformed themselves into limiting, though comfortably familiar perspectives, attitudes and patterns. They were all a part of me, so extensively imbedded that I didn't know they might or could be separated out.

As examples, our attitudes and perspectives about worthiness, about the appropriateness of various feelings, and the very nature of the world in which we live are established quite early in life. A great deal of this "truth" is defined by the adults we have known as children and by our interpretation and feelings evoked by what they said and did. Without meaning to, parents perpetuate this process, passing on to their young or to children in their charge what they, themselves, once learned. Obviously this can be both advantageous and harmful. We all tend to spend our adult lives rerunning the equivalent of these old hard drive computer programs, some of which are invaluable to us, and others which we did not consciously create or necessarily want. All the same, we tend to recreate the emotional environment, to stay in that place which is familiar, regardless of how destructive or limiting it might be.

This is a true story, a real adventure about discovery. Among other things, it explores the process of loosening the chains.

I have a dear old Chinese friend in Hong Kong who is a healer, a wise man and a Chinese herbalist. On Tuesday mornings I used to meet Dr. Wu with his interpreter at one of the local teahouses while they chain-smoked and had their dim sum breakfast. One of my questions for him was this:

"Dr. Wu, I think that since I have asked for and allowed more joy in my life it is helping me to get well. Do you think this is true?"

He responded for several minutes in Cantonese, which eventually produced three English sentences. "Joy is extremely important; but if the joy is like a blanket, covering over old misery, it won't help. It will only be temporary. The important part of my answer to you is to get rid of the misery in your life."

That is what I did. I worked hard to chip away at inauthenticity, at being less than true to myself, and at healing or withdrawing from relationships which had been harmful. "Shoulds" were replaced by "coulds,"

2

and I began to look out for myself. With other phenomenal experiences and divine help, the healing began to kick in, and my physical condition turned around.

I came upon healing realms, which were not only unknown to me, but also unimaginable. I explored them all. In this way this book is a true adventure story. Cancer was the catalyst, pressing me to the choice: shall I stand here like the elephant with the rope around me and give up? Or consider trying a different way and hope to be well again?

This is not a "how to" book—the journey was tailor made, as is everyone's; but there are basic elements which will be useful to many people. While the disease pressed me to explore and develop, it eventually became far less important than what I was able to discover about life and about living. This is, therefore, not a book which is intended exclusively for people who are ill. It illuminates for the healthy as well, the strength of the human spirit and the dangers of chains and inauthenticity.

"If the head and body are to be well," Plato wrote, "you must begin by curing the soul; that is the first thing...the great error of our day in the treatment of the human body [is] that physicians separate the soul from the body." This disunion described eons ago has been the attitude and perspective for much of Western medicine today.

In this book I do not reject traditional medicine, but believe that it needs to be redefined as one component of healing. In my situation, traditional Western medicine bought me time in which to develop a personal healing approach. In this light, and without question, it helped me to begin to save my life. Standing alone, however, the technology, the chemicals and the great gifts of my excellent doctors, could not have done it alone.

To hold a broader relevance, traditional Western medicine needs to move away from its dogmatic, sometimes arrogant stance. Within the relatively short period of time spent writing this book, it seems to be happening. In truth, a partnership, another industry, has already begun to form; a partnership which recognizes that healing involves the mind and spirit as well as the body. This linkage is being forged by a collection of brave pioneering doctors, by patients and by their loved ones. Every year an increasing number of medical schools, much aware of the success and popularity of this renewed direction, have chosen to pursue a more inclusive approach.

In the final analysis this is a story which gives hope.

1

If the only tool you possess is a hammer,
You will see the world as a collection of nails.

—Anonymous

This story doesn't actually begin with the man who sat next to me at lunch, but he is my doorway into the telling of it.

It was 1990. My husband, Geoff, and I were in London on our way to the annual Rowing Regatta at Henley-upon-Thames. The stranger we were scheduled to meet had traveled from America to see one of his children. Mutual friends had suggested that we get together to share our unusual travel experiences. We were all a little pressed for time, but we agreed to meet for lunch at Claridge's Hotel in Mayfair.

He was an intelligent looking man with an easy smile and wild eyebrows, which seemed to meander this way and that across the upper part of his face. His bearing and clothes were academic. The world he respected was made up of facts and figures. Once we had ordered lunch he began to share his vast collection: heights of mountains in various parts of the world, population figures, economic growth in places we had visited over the years. There were new rice crop yields in The Philippines and inflated hotel prices in Italy. Numbers were this man's passion. I wondered if he was with the U.N. or possibly The Ford Foundation.

In most English circles it is not considered polite to speak of one's profession. Geoff finally couldn't stand it any longer, and American-to-American he asked.

"I am an oncologist," the man replied, "a cancer doctor." There was a perceptible pause in which Geoff and I did not look at one another.

My short hair had only just grown back. Two weeks before, two blonde wigs had been tossed into the Hong Kong jungle for birds to use as nests. I had been dealing with cancer myself, and had come to associate the medical world with the odds makers: Drs. Jimmy-the-Greek.

I had had surgery to remove two lymphoma tumors from my abdominal area; there was liver involvement, but bone marrow was "clean." A rigorous course of chemotherapy followed, as well as many extraordinary experiences in the realm of healing. Neither Geoff nor I were about to tell this man about any of it. Mine was a private story. It was still young, in need of protection and strengthening before it could stand up before someone as cool and detached as this.

At the time of our meeting I knew intuitively that remnants of the disease lingered on. My self-confidence and beliefs were being tested; it was a delicate time.

Having been asked about his work, the oncologist rose to the occasion with great aplomb.

"I am very discouraged;" he said, lowering his voice to a level of intimate pontification; "chemotherapy has not produced the results we had hoped for. The cure rate really is very low, you know, and the problem is that when the cure is less than complete, the chemotherapy itself can trigger new cancers. We've got to attack it in another way. What we are doing is just not good enough."

His speech was terrifying. Geoff was quiet. He was leaving the response to me. I tried to turn the conversation to a more hopeful direction.

"But there are other dimensions to the healing process. Have you read any of the books which deal with the importance of the patient's attitude? The value of meditation and the untapped healing energy inside all of us? I have just finished an especially good book by an East Indian doctor, [Deepak Chopra], who has a clinic outside of Boston..."

"Quacks!" he interrupted, turning his chin to one side and quickly back again. "There are so many quacks out there now. Money-hungry wolves preying on the ignorant, desperate public."

"But what you have said is true: the best that Western Medicine has to offer isn't enough. I worked in Medical Research while Geoff was in Business School."

"What were you looking at?" the doctor asked.

"I was gathering data for a radiologist on a population of adults who had had their thymus glands irradiated when they were children. There was a lot of interest 50 years ago in the thymus gland and its possible role in Crib Death."

"What did your group find?"

"We found that the Study Group had more common colds. Actually our work didn't yield anything significant, but my point is that people are always looking for better healing odds."

"They always are. But their search won't come to anything," he said. "They are not looking in the right places. These other methods need to be scientifically proven. Solutions have to be found in the real world."

"Who is defining what the real world is?" I asked in silence.

Hedging this heavy discussion, the doctor cocked his head to one side.

"C'mon," he said, "this other stuff is airy fairy business. All nonsense. And the worst ones!" he said, trying to strengthen his case, "I'll tell you who they are: those so-called Psychic Healers in The Philippines. They are real frauds, every last one of them!" The eyebrows were really moving now, and his chin rose to make the point. "I saw one once, working in Baguio. The village people moved me to the front to watch when they found out I was a doctor. Well, it is a criminal deception! It is magic and trickery, nothing more. What they claim to do is quite impossible."

After a short pause, Geoff had the good sense to ask for the check. We finished our coffee and said good-bye.

In the privacy of the cab, we were quietly numb, sitting there cloaked in silence, staring blankly at the outside world. Finally the driver asked where we would like to go. Moving deeper into the anonymity of the flowing traffic, tears ran down my cheeks.

Geoff put his big, loving arms around me and they came faster. The kindly London cabby softened his driving style, and we made our way back to Cadogan Gardens in the little black cocoon.

I thought about my healing miracles, some dramatic, some subtle. This man dismissed them as coincidences, frauds, and "airy fairy nonsense." These incredible building blocks of healing were condemned by the omniscient arrogance of the scientific method.

This doctor looked at people as pieces of machinery, treating their symptoms without understanding the relationship between physical illness and the other significant aspects of human life, such as personality, perspective on life, family situation, and lifestyle. He seemed to know very little apart from his numbers; yet there he sat, in a powerful place of authority influencing the lives, and deaths, of his patients. In the end I realized that my tears were for them, for faces never seen.

Driving to the theatre later that evening, as the cozy glow of London's dusk bathed its silhouetted rooftops, I talked to our youngest child about this meeting. Her response was clear and removed all residual sadness.

"You know, Mamita," she said, her nine-year-old face radiant, "people who haven't been born yet will look back on us as primitives. With what they will know even 100 years from now, it will be like looking back on cavemen. We're not so advanced, but, you know, sometimes we act as though we are the smartest people who will ever live."

It is that simple. I am certain that the reality we serve is far less powerful than the reality just beyond. Our thoughts and attitudes are extremely important; they create the future and either bring about or exclude new possibilities in our lives. I know that love, the transformation of destructive patterns and memories, and ultimate forgiveness, are the keys to positive growth and healing. Being in touch with our feelings and honoring them enhances a life with lightness; and storing misery, perhaps in the form of resentment or hurt, knowingly or inadvertently, can make us as sick as a Love Canal can.

I also know that there aren't any roadmaps to this land of miracles. It is a journey we make alone, surrendering the illusion of control in our lives, selecting teachers and reading signposts along the way. We combine inner listening with personal responsibility for our choices. Often through suffering we are led to surrender, to listen and trust our instincts, and in doing so, to develop a rare type of responsibility and courage.

My miracles, everyone's miracles, are natural occurrences. They will seem wonderfully ordinary in the reality just beyond, in the New Frontier of the Twenty-First Century. This story is about my entry into the territory, which we, as a culture, have only begun to explore.

2

A pebble dropped into a pool awakens sleeping encirclements.

—L.S. Peters, 1959

Events take on a different meaning when we look at them with hindsight. It is in the backward glance that they become warnings, indicators of bumps in the road, or validations of paths already chosen.

Three summers before our trip to London I had an experience, which began as something of a lark, but later could be seen as prophetic.

From a fairly conventional arena of life, I had chosen to do something bold and bizarre. An especially dear friend arranged for me to see a clairvoyant in Beverly, Massachusetts. It seems unremarkable now, as psychics or mediums can be reached by dialing a 1-900 telephone number, but making a secretive foray into such an unknown world at that time, was for me nothing less than adventuresome. Conventional people didn't do such things; if they did, they would keep it to themselves.

The young woman I went to see turned out to be lovely. In a still photograph she would have been very prosaic-looking, but on running footage she had a beautiful luminosity which, when combined with her integrity, was disarming.

I remember using her bathroom and feeling comforted by the fact that it was impeccably clean. (Clean bathrooms always indicated a certain level of well-placed values.) Her apartment was festooned with hanging plants, all of them healthy (another good sign), and with large canvases of East Indian cotton. The sun shone brightly through the windows and onto polished blonde wooden floors.

Once we settled down the young medium explained that she was going to meditate and then give me information about my life. I was to sit there quietly and relax. Relaxing, it seemed, might be difficult. Her information was specific in nature. In many ways it was the overture for the drama to follow. The first point she made was quite interesting.

"There are two countries which you and your husband should try to live in," she said. "What is your husband's name?"

"Geoffrey. Geoff."

"You and Geoff should make an effort to live in Japan and India." After a short pause, "If you can't actually live there, try to take an extended vacation in each place. And do it before you are old."

The young woman had my attention. It was uncanny. Geoff had received a traveling fellowship through Harvard College, and as newlyweds we had spent the better part of a year in India. More recently we had lived in Tokyo, where he had set up a securities sales activity for a Wall Street investment bank. It was uncanny.

But if the young woman was gifted enough to see the significance of these two countries in our lives, why didn't she know we had already lived there? And why did she need to ask Geoff's name?

"We have lived in both of these countries already," I told her. "We just left Tokyo at the beginning of the summer to move to Hong Kong."

"Good," she said, nonplused neither by our "coincidence" nor by her not knowing.

When I asked about our three children, about Geoff, my sister, parents, and parents-in-law, her information was extremely specific; her knowledge of events known only to me was incredible. Her tone was even and forthright.

"Your daughter has had a serious illness within the past couple of years. Something in her backbone."

"Yes," I said. "She had osteomyelitis. She was in the Mass General Hospital for nearly three months."

"She is fine now, but while she was ill she was deciding whether she wanted to stay or leave."

"Leave what? Do you mean whether she wanted to live or die?"

"Yes. Whether or not she wanted to leave the planet."

There was a large box of Kleenex on the table. I took one. I wanted to know more about the children, where they were going, and what I could do to help them along their way.

"Your children are very talented and beautiful," she said. "Your older ones will be successful in The Arts, and your youngest one is a very bright light. She came in at a special time and she will do good things; she will help the planet, possibly as a lawyer. She is definitely an achiever. They all are. You have taken great care with your children."

I asked for explanations of behavior in others, which I had found difficult. In her opinion these patterns were usually linked to past lives.

"They continue the pattern until they choose to change it. It isn't your problem unless you accept responsibility for them."

This was a stretch for my understanding, but it was possible to take vague comfort in what she had to say.

Then she added, "You and your husband had important lives in Japan and India. You were in charge of a large monastery in Japan, and Geoff was a holy man in India."

The session slipped into comic relief as I pictured Geoff in a pin-striped loincloth with matted hair and a face with red and white sacred paint. But was it a coincidence that we had lived in both of these countries? Were we led unknowingly to these places like little wind-up toys?

Toward the end of the session, she said, "Why don't you ask about yourself?"

"I know most of what I need to know about myself."

"No, you don't."

"Then what do I need to know?"

She paused, her eyes still closed. "You have a very beautiful aura," she said. "There aren't any black or dark spots. You have clarity and integrity. You are quite a strong woman. You have a great sense of humor which often saves you from getting stuck in the mud, and you have a lot on your shoulders."

"I don't know anything about auras, but I would like to think that I'm all right. In the fine tuning, I have plenty of things to work on, but the basics are probably OK."

The young woman went quiet for what seemed like a long time. Was the session over?

"While your aura is beautiful, it is very, very weak." She reached for the glass on a small side table and drank some water. "You are giving yourself, your life away, your joyous energy. You are giving it away to your husband, your children, to difficult relatives and to friends. I also see a school. You spend too much time looking after it. The best way to describe what is happening is to say that you are over-spending yourself."

"Is that a bad thing?" I argued. "What could be wrong with it? Most of it feels good to me, and isn't it true that in giving we also receive? I was brought up to be like this, to look after everybody."

"You are giving too much without replenishing your own energy. I am telling you that you are seriously weak. Selflessness is a foolish and misguided concept. It can be dangerous."

"How can you tell that I am weak?"

"Your aura is diluted. The buttercup yellow color, or hue, is beautiful, but extremely muted. Why don't you take care of yourself?"

"But I do! I jog three times a week; I spend time with good friends and with the children; I have fulfilling projects going all the time. I eat well, and try to get enough sleep."

"But you never relax," she insisted. Take more time for your emotional needs, and for your spiritual development. You should be further along than you are."

"Further along where?" I wondered.

"Develop your art work."

She opened her eyes for the first time since the session had begun.

"Do you meditate?" she asked.

"No."

"Why not?"

"It isn't a comfortable idea for me."

"Why?"

"Because I think it might be anti-Christian."

"But you do have great success with prayer," she said.

"Yes, in fact I do." Amazing.

"Well, prayer is a form of meditation."

"It is?"

"Of course it is. Learn to meditate as soon as you can, and do it every day. Make time for it; quiet time just for you. Ten minutes to start, then try to increase it to 20 or 30. I'm telling you: you have to pay attention and replenish yourself. Find out what your emotional needs are and honor them. Then encourage your husband and children to honor them. They don't know that you have any needs. It isn't their fault; for a number of reasons you have hidden this from them. Look into it. And try to find a Japanese way of meditating. It will suit you best."

A Japanese way.

I registered the advice and said I would try.

The young woman's eyes fixed on mine with a firm intensity.

"Look," she said, "please do what I am telling you. You will be in trouble if you don't. Look at your life carefully. Scrutinize the relationships; look at the marriage you have. None of them are good for you as they are. You are allowing yourself to be held responsible for too much, and no one is taking care of you, not even yourself."

The hour was up. I paid the young woman her fee, and said goodbye with thanks.

It was all very interesting. I would have to think about it for a while. Yes, I would think about it.

3

I did not arrive at my understanding of the fundamental laws of the universe through my rational mind.

—Albert Einstein

The following autumn we returned to Hong Kong, to our house on The Peak. It is quite a good house, with generously proportioned rooms and plenty of light, but as often happens on the hills in Hong Kong, the actual house is incidental. The view is everything. Tucked into the side of a rambling green hillside, it looks out and over a vast expanse of The South China Sea. Here, an endless flow of ships from places far away pass through, always bringing stories with them, hundreds of stories of adventure and intrigue. More than six million travelers from all over the world made their way to Hong Kong each year in those times, and I would guess that most of them made it a point of getting up to The Peak to click their cameras on a clear day.

In the mornings the air is alive with the activity of birds, hundreds of birds, and the soft rustling sounds of swaying bamboo. By late afternoon the falling sun plays exotically on the water's surface, giving it a gossamer quality, with vibrant, shimmering gold and silver. And the nights! I will never forget them. Mysteriously foggy or glamorously clear, the ships were always there, illuminated by warm yellow running lights; at other times cloaked in clouds giving off the deeply resonant warning of their horns: "We are here. Take care. We are here."

After several weeks had passed I was driving home, up The Peak Road, when an advertisement came over the radio for The Vital Life Centre in Central. This was the place from which to follow "New Age" interests. The advertisement nudged my memory, and I wrote down the telephone number.

A few days later I telephoned.

"Is there anyone there who can teach me how to meditate?" I asked.

The query dropped with a thud and the line was silent. I became self-conscious and uncertain about this new direction and was tempted to hang up the receiver.

Then the founder of the Center, Nancy Beckor, came on the line.

"Hello," she said. "What sort of meditation are you interested in?" By her accent, she was Australian.

"I don't know enough about it to answer. I was wondering if you could help me."

"Why don't you start by coming in for a Reiki Treatment?" Nancy suggested.

"What is that?" I asked. "Is it Icelandic?" (From Reykjavik. It seemed a logical guess.)

"No," she said, laughing. "It is a form of meditation which enhances spiritual growth and promotes physical healing. It is Japanese."

Japanese. I took the first available appointment.

When the day came, I made my way to The Vital Life Centre. Nancy was gently enthusiastic, attractive and professional. She was also focused, with a lot of commercial responsibility on her shoulders. We shared an admiration for Issey Miyake clothes, and in typical Hong Kong style, compared notes on sewing ladies who could copy them inexpensively and well.

Nancy ushered me into one of the small treatment rooms, motioned for me to sit down beside her desk, and handed me a file card. On the line marked "Reason for Reiki Treatment:" I answered simply, "Meditation."

There was a massage table in the room, as well as a stool. At Nancy's instruction I took off my shoes and wristwatch and lay down on my back.

"Now," she said, "close your eyes and try to keep your mind clear of any thoughts: a blank inner screen. No shopping lists, business plans, no problem solving. You can go to sleep if you like, but please relax completely."

I nodded.

As she washed her hands she continued, "I will play a tape of quieting music, mostly to drown out the traffic noise in the street."

The room lights were turned off and the music clicked on in the cassette player. Dim light filtered through the metal blinds; while trying to relax I wondered uneasily about what would happen next.

Nancy placed her hands just above my face, on either side of my nose. Even though she didn't actually touch me, there was a wondrously soft and comforting warmth, which seemed to flow from her palms. It was like nothing I had ever felt before in its soothing smoothness. After a few minutes she moved on to another part of my head. There would be nine more "positions" before the basic treatment would be complete.

13

(These are generally done in a specific sequence, beginning either at the head or above the waist. In an emergency, however, a Reiki practitioner begins to work immediately on the area in need of healing.)

At the third position, the excitement began. As Nancy cradled the back of my head in her hands, eyes still closed and mind quiet, I began to see vibrant colors, as though they were being projected onto a motion picture screen. First there was a vibrant periwinkle blue in round shapes. It looked as though an electric light was shining through from behind. This soon expanded and became the background for two very bright yellow circles, which appeared in the middle, side-by-side, like a Peter Max cartoon of two fried eggs. The yellow circles would diminish and disappear; then they would come back a moment later and become two full circles again. This happened repeatedly. It was absolutely thrilling to watch, particularly as I had no idea where it all came from. I lay there smiling with amazement.

When Nancy moved on to the abdominal area, another phenomenon was added in the form of the terrific, burning heat which came through her hands. It was almost too hot to be comfortable. What did it mean? Was this a good sign or a bad one?

After that the rest of the Reiki Treatment was quiet and comparatively uneventful. Eventually I did fall into a short, blissfully deep sleep, waking up feeling refreshed and balanced. It was very special, like nothing I had ever experienced.

"That was amazing," I said later, struggling to hook my watchband.

"Reiki *is* amazing," Nancy replied.

"I saw this beautiful bright periwinkle blue and yellow. What does that mean?"

"What you saw was energy."

"Does this happen to everyone who has a Reiki Treatment?"

"No, not to everyone. It was some kind of message that you were given, but I can't tell you what it means."

"Why can't you?"

"Because I don't know."

"Then what good is it?"

"It will become clear later. You will see. The part that concerns me is the intense heat in your stomach around the solar plexus."

Is that where the solar plexus is? I had often wondered.

"I was worried that it might be burning you. Did it hurt your hands?"

"No," Nancy assured me. "I can feel the heat channeling through me, but it never burns. It is divine energy. I am just the vehicle. You were receiving all that I could pass on in the abdomen. There is a definite problem there. Have you seen a medical doctor?"

"Yes. I have been seeing British doctors for more than a year now, but they can't seem to come up with anything. My digestive tract hasn't been right for a while."

"Why didn't you mention this when you were filling out the card?"

"I honestly didn't think it was important. So far the doctors think it is some sort of parasite or infection. It often happens in this part of the world. I struggled with a bug in India for months once and eventually got so thin that my wedding rings fell off, but I hadn't thought of this as anything to worry about."

"Well, you need to pay attention. Get to the bottom of this as soon as you can," Nancy said. "Change doctors if you have to."

We said good-bye and I stopped at the desk to make another appointment for two weeks later.

I did change physicians. There were more tests, more pills and more dead ends. Weeks and months passed and there was no change. Could it be a rare intestinal worm from China or Thailand? Or a new virus from Southern China, the virus capitol of the world? (Viruses breed and mutate in the duck population there.) The mystery continued; the doctors didn't seem to be worried, so neither was I.

Meanwhile, Reiki treatments became a bi-monthly routine. The vibrant colors persisted and the heat in the solar plexus was constant, but less intense. Periwinkle blue and yellow always appeared in varying forms. Sometimes there were dots of yellow pussywillows appearing and dissolving on a periwinkle ground. Other times there were beckoning tunnels to walk through. The tunnels were a soft and comforting shade of baby blue. As time went on, more colors came: bright vermilion and pink, then a deep purple surrounded with white light. The "messages" were piling up, as was my personal frustration for not being able to understand them. But the two Peter Max fried eggs recurred repeatedly and were the most compelling.

These experiences were invigorating, and tweaked a curiosity and appetite for metaphysical adventures. However, they didn't seem to lead anywhere. There was a great show, and then nothing until the next great show. What was the point of it? Who or what was playing games with me?

By the time Spring came, I was overtaken by frustration. Nancy told me to be patient.

"Trust the timing," she would say.

"But you don't understand. My suitcases are packed and I am ready to go, but I don't know where."

"Relax. Trust. Let it happen."

"I'm tired of waiting. I want a roadmap. I want to understand the colors and to at least know where I am being directed."

At Nancy's suggestion I attended the Reiki I Healing Seminar given by a Swiss Master who had just been with the Dalai Lama in New Delhi.

Reiki is an ancient healing method, which actually traces its origins to Tibet. From there it mysteriously disappeared, surfacing in Japan centuries later. Some historians believe that Jesus visited Tibet. If so, it is quite possible that he was introduced to Reiki there. It is also possible that he was born with this particular gift.

The Japanese Kanji for Reiki is: 靈
氣

In simple terms it means "spiritually-guided energy." It is guided by God, and can never be used to do harm.

The seminar in Hong Kong provided instruction in the history of Reiki, as well as hands-on practice. In the attuning process, the palm, crown and heart chakras are opened by the Reiki Master; afterwards one feels noticeably changed. Within the first day it was easy to feel the wondrous flow of heat from my hands and an intimacy with its source.

After an initial exposure to Reiki in Hong Kong I gave myself a treatment on awakening every morning, as well as sporadically throughout the day.

In addition to the Reiki I Seminar, Nancy suggested that I attend "An Evening with Lazaris."

A man named Jack Purcell allows a spirit entity called Lazaris (pronounced La-ZAR-us), to speak through him. Lazaris talks about the conscious choices we need to make to reach a state of fulfillment in our lives. He describes the tools of creation: desire, imagination and expectancy, and combines them with pragmatic good sense. He pokes a bit of fun at The Human Potential Movement, suggesting that the only potential we need is within ourselves. This appealed to me.

He was extremely interesting, but I wasn't ready to move into this arena. Lazaris was from a different world, beyond my understanding or inclination.

When summer came, we left Hong Kong for America. The doctors had yet to figure out what was wrong with me. It was probably nothing.

4

Coincidences are God's way of remaining anonymous.

—Quoted by Dr. Bernie Siegel in
Love, Medicine & Miracles

June, July and August of 1989 passed in a fluid dream. In the Sierra Mountains in California, time meanders and then eventually gives up trying to assert itself. The days become full and round and one loses one's sense of linear, segmented time.

Completing conversations with a sense of satisfaction became more important than keeping to a schedule. As a family we laughed more, slept longer and thrived blissfully in the mountain air. When good friends came to stay, they, too, were infected with this carefree feeling. It was a summer of long, late breakfasts, trail rides and rodeos, bathed in high country sunlight, and picnics by boat. In the minty shadows, one could take refuge from the sun and smell the pine and lupine.

It seemed to me that on that vacation we were all beginning to realize the need to rearrange our lives, giving more thought to easy-going times.

Wrapped in a Chinese silk duvet, I liked best to watch the arrival of the new day from the pier. A layer of subtle pink and mauve and purple would precede the arrival of the giant fireball. Once the sun began to creep over the mountaintops it seemed to be virtually hurled into the sky, leaving the peaks a brilliant yellow with soft light radiating from behind. Once the day was born, I would quietly creep back into the house, go back to bed and sleep again.

My digestive tract was still not right. I seemed to eat less. By August I began to lose a little weight, but I was riding twice a week, doing exercises to increase the power in my upper thighs. The goal was to be able to gallop with my legs, arms raised in the air.

In late August the spell ended. Suitcases were packed, dustcovers spread over the furniture, refrigerator cleaned, and the fireplace closed with a wooden board. Grouchy and silent, we loaded the car and returned to the real world. First stop: San Francisco.

The children had medical examinations, dental appointments, and haircuts, and then there were last-minute school needs. There were hugs and farewell tears; finally everyone flew off in different directions to begin the academic year. Geoff flew back to Hong Kong with our little one. The two older children headed for schools on the East Coast, and I stayed behind for two days with my parents. It was a well-earned respite, two days of quiet, purposeful, but slower.

On the first night, Mother prepared a special Scandinavian pork roast. We had a wonderful evening, but I went off to bed feeling a bit peculiar. Perhaps the food had been a little rich. (After living in Japan our diets had moved away from pork and beef to chicken, fish and vegetables.)

By early morning, I was violently ill. Curled up in a ball on the carpet in the bathroom, afraid to leave the proximity of the loo, it was cold and I was scared for the first time. Even then, I vaguely clung to organizing skills, and wondered if the return to Hong Kong might be delayed. Fortunately there was an annual doctor's appointment scheduled for the next day.

The following morning I was on the examining table telling the older doctor about the previous night. On probing he found a lump in the abdominal area. He had been concerned when he examined the same place last year. "Let's watch this," he had said. "Something funny is going on here."

This time he said, "You'll need to see a surgeon about this." He had someone specific in mind, and reached for the telephone. With his hand over the receiver he said, "We might not be able to get an appointment on such short notice."

"Who is the surgeon you want me to see?" I asked.

"The Bay Area's best: Bob Albo."

In the chain of divine events, Bob Albo was not only the Bay Area's best, he was also a friend.

"We are neighbors at the lake," I said.

I was given an appointment within the hour.

Geoff was already in Hong Kong, so my younger sister, Cindy, drove me to Dr. Albo's office.

As the nurse called me in I thought, "It's a hernia. I'll bet it's a hernia."

We talked about summer at the lake and about the drought. Everyone had his or her fingers crossed, hoping for a heavy winter snowfall. Then Dr. Albo looked at the lab work and moved me onto an elevated chair for the physical exam. He was concerned and masterful, and assured me in a very comforting way that we would have answers as soon as possible.

"Is it a hernia?" I asked, playing the old wish one more time.

"Could be." He probed and palpated round and round in the same place. By his tone and pause in answering, I could tell that a hernia was not at the top of his list.

Bob ordered a sonogram, gave me a hug, and sent us to the hospital. It was a hot Indian Summer's day. There were slices of cool watermelon, bouquets of wild flowers and picnic baskets on the cover of the *Sunset* magazine, but summer was over. There was nothing carefree about this.

The technician was very chatty.

"This looks fine," she would say, again and again, as she moved the sonogram over my baby-oiled tummy. "I don't see any problem here."

When I had worked at The Massachusetts General Hospital in Boston, technicians were not allowed to offer their opinions; but in this case it was good to hear what she had to say. I sank down into a feeling of comfortable, sweet relief. I would just be a day or so late in getting back to Hong Kong.

When I was dressed and ready to leave, a radiologist came out from one of the cubbyholes.

"It doesn't look good," he said.

"What is it?" I asked.

"You will have to speak to Dr. Albo."

No, I thought to myself, I want to speak to you. I would like to know now.

I resurrected terms from medical research days and attempted to position myself in the inner circle where communication might follow less rigid rules and guidelines.

"It looks like a lymphoma tumor. Dr. Albo will probably order a C-T Scan for tomorrow, early."

The rest of the words never reached me. Behind the veil of disbelief was a vision of Edvard Munch's woodprint called "The Scream." It was a horrific scream, which no one else could hear. To me, it sounded like a field full of cicadas, crying out in chorus on a hot day. I was transported to a place where time is frozen and the silence is petrifying.

Putting my head on the unknown doctor's shoulder, all I could manage was, "Oh no."

After a few moments he asked me why I didn't cry, but I couldn't answer.

I went back to the waiting room, sat down beside Cindy and kept looking straight ahead. Our first communication was a thumbs down signal. A full two minutes later I passed on the news. The frozen message began to thaw and move into reality. Still there weren't any tears.

The C-T Scan on Friday verified the preliminary diagnosis. Again we were in Dr. Albo's office.

"It's bad news, Sweetie Pie," he said, "but it's the very best of bad news. It's a lymphoma tumor and it's got to come out right away."

I asked, "How soon?"

"Right away."

"But tomorrow is Saturday."

"I'll do it for you early in the morning."

We sat together for a few moments, talked about the logistics, and then I asked, "Can I ask you a favor?"

"Sure," Bob answered. "What is it?"

"Will you ask your OR Team to be careful of what they say while I am under anesthesia? I don't want to subconsciously hear them discussing or speculating on my situation, especially if it looks difficult. It could sabotage the healing."

"I will see to it. I have a very good team."

"Good," I said. "I think it is important."

I wondered to myself, I do? Where did this idea come from?

There was another hug and more words of encouragement.

As we drove home a distant lightbulb turned on in my head. The young woman in Massachusetts. Had she seen this coming and had she tried to warn me? What else had she talked about? Depleted energy and a weak aura, what else?

5

Cancer is a symbol, as most illness is, of something going wrong in the patient's life, warning him to take another road.

—Elida Evans, *Psychological Study of Cancers,* 1926

The surgery was carried out early the next day. When I woke up, one of the first of many, innumerable kindnesses awaited me. A bookstore owner in Marin County had given Cindy a set of audiotapes of Dr. Bernie Siegel reading from his book, *Love, Medicine, and Miracles.* Cindy had asked her advice on which books to purchase, and this lovely lady tossed in the set of Bernie Siegel cassettes, which had helped her get through her own experience of cancer.

"Bernie Siegel is *my* present," she had said. "He will get your sister off on the right foot."

Bernie Siegel was a godsend. From the second post-operative day I would lie down with the Walkman, close my eyes and listen to this wise and wonderful man. When the tape was over, I would push PLAY again. In and out of groggy sleep, the positive messages were heard by the sub-conscious, laying important groundwork for healing. When family members or friends would call, it took a little time to undo the headset. My standard answer was, "Sorry, it took me a minute to get the phone. I was in bed with Bernie Siegel." With tubes running in and out of my body and surgical staple train tracks across my abdomen, it seemed a patheti-cally acceptable joke. Besides, a good sense of humor is something Bernie Siegel encourages in his patients. I felt he wouldn't mind.

Through these tapes I learned that it was necessary to stay spirited and feisty. Passive, good little patients don't fare as well. "Keep your power," Bernie would say; "keep your identity." He gave me the confi-dence to accept the benefits of Western Medicine while looking with hope beyond its limiting aspects. This is an extraordinary gift.

Everything Dr. Siegel said made sense. He reminded me that I was a human being with dreams yet to fulfill, plans to pursue, and things to look forward to. And I was never, never to allow anyone to treat me as a statistic.

On one tape, he tells the story of a patient who wants to live and see her eldest son married. Having made it to the wedding, she returns to Dr. Siegel and says, "By the way, I have two more sons."

"Healing occurs for reasons that medical schools don't understand," Dr. Siegel insists. I have since learned that there aren't many medical statistics on so-called miraculous healings, because patients who experience them generally do not report them to their doctors.

There are many stories in the healing world of patients augmenting their traditional treatments with healing herbs, homeopathic remedies, energy work, yoga and focused meditation. If a patient is helped, the doctor might express surprise or annoyance. He might say, "This is impossible. It has been proven that 'X' doesn't work." The average patient takes these remarks to heart, accepts the "expert's" truth, and begins to regress.

Newspapers can also be culprits in sabotaging the healing process. Again, Bernie Siegel describes a patient who had been improving remarkably on a regime of laetrile, when after several months, he read in the newspaper that laetrile didn't work. His healing immediately reversed itself and he died. Again, this individual had replaced his own unfolding truth, his own belief, with someone else's, with dire results.

What does this tell us about the power of thought and what we allow into our consciousness? And how much power should we give to the "experts"?

Bernie Siegel reminds us that we are in charge of our own case. The doctors are not. The doctors would therefore work for me, ideally *with* me. I have choices; if I don't like a doctor's manner or attitude, I can replace him with another. This is exceedingly important to understand. We cannot behave like Konrad Lorenz's fledgling goslings who, on hatching from their eggs, follow the first moving creature in a position of authority they see.

I had a dear friend In Hong Kong who was diagnosed with an extremely rare and terminal disease. His doctor in London told him point blank that the disease was incurable and that he had less than six months to live. My even-tempered friend raised his voice and prolonged his life considerably.

"Don't ever assume to call my case incurable," he said. "What you mean is that *you* don't know how to cure me, and that is a very different matter."

His doctor apparently smiled and eventually learned what a terminally ill patient can do to claim his power and extend his life. My friend lived well for six years.

Along with the Siegel tapes, there was a room full of flowers from friends and family well-wishers. Not another miracle? It felt like one. I was benefiting from sustained prayers and positive thoughts, from their weekly telephone calls, books, and from videos which were sent. One came from a good friend who performs in a Stand-Up Comedy Club in New York City and another from the school I had been affiliated with in Japan. These gifts, among many, many others, enhanced enormously the healing-prone environment.

After the first two weeks I could feel the love of friends and family encircling me like a galvanized fence, strong and firm and constant. This is what people arguing with a disease need to feel, love and connection from all, including the unexpected directions, from close friends as well as others they might have lost track of, old neighbors and colleagues. There is a transformation to grace, which, in critical times, moves human beings beyond kindness. The loving energy is powerful enough to commune with. I was to learn later that one of the primary aspects of healing is the feeling of connectedness we have with one another, and with all living things. This realization is experiential and life altering.

After the surgery, Geoff and I agreed to tell our two older children about what we were going through. Lex, our daughter, was on a special program on the Island of Kalymnos in Greece. She didn't have a telephone and was impossible to reach. But Peter was at school in Massachusetts. I called the headmaster, explained the situation, and we arranged to talk with Peter later in the day.

"Hi, Mom. What's going on? Everyone is acting weird here. It's creepy. Has something happened to Dad?"

"No, Sweetie. It's me. I have hit a snag. I won't be going back to Hong Kong for a while."

"Why? What is it?"

It was a slow conversation, first brave, then vulnerable, and tough going for both of us. It was terrible to deliver such news without being there to touch and hold one another. I worried that Peter felt alone and scared, so the conversation was infused with as much optimism as I could muster.

Peter listened, and then in a cracking voice he said,

"You know how much I love you, and I hate to think of you

suffering, but I think this is going to be good for our family. We're all out of whack. You know we are. I know we are. Everybody will pay attention now. It is your turn to be taken care of. But for me to be right, you have to beat this thing."

This intuitive, loving response from a sixteen-year-old, brave and hopeful, matched the feelings I had not been able to put into words. The rest of the day was spent in and out of tears. My feelings had been blurred by the surprise of it all, by the fear of the unknown, and strangely enough, by simply stepping up to the task. Peter's comments were a reminder to look at the patterns of our family and my own. We reluctantly said good-bye and agreed to talk often.

Before leaving the hospital, one of Bernie Siegel's lessons came up for review. A middle-aged radiologist came into my room to give his evaluation while Geoff was there. It seemed like a thoughtful, positive gesture. He was a pleasant man, and talked non-stop in a lecturing style for about 10 minutes, outlining the probabilities and options, including the statistics of my case.

His information was serious and interesting and scary. There were numbers and percentages and odds. Upon finishing, he took a deep, resuscitating breath, stepped off of his stage and seemed to mentally switch channels. He leaned back in the chair and shifted his body toward Geoff.

"Well," he said, "it must be interesting living in Hong Kong now. What's your opinion of 1997 and the Chinese takeover there?"

Geoff, who is definitely a task-oriented person, began to answer, but I interrupted. My voice was even and straightforward.

"You have just spent 10 minutes describing a disease that is threatening my life. It's my *life*. I could die from this. Don't you want to know if I have any questions or reactions to what you've said?"

"Yes. Of course."

Geoff and I had other meetings with the doctors who were immediately involved. Important decisions were made. With liver involvement, chemotherapy was the place to start. We agreed to it. It would be a very aggressive course, administered every 21 days, provided that the white blood count was adequate.

There was another development to deal with from a different direction. Geoff announced to me one October afternoon that he had decided to quit his job, one that he had enjoyed enormously, and considered the high point of his Wall Street career.

How abundant life is with ironies. In the loving partnership we formed 25 years before, we had chosen a lifestyle in which professional fulfillment and then financial success would take precedence, at least for a while, over other important aspects of life. In support of the extensive demands on Geoff's professional time, I had taken care of everyone and everything outside of work. I protected him from problems and crises, took over all lines of family communication, and without intending to, contributed to his inclination to become a serious workaholic. This was not an unusual pattern in the professional arena we occupied. Misguided, well-meaning folly had led us to this place together, but leaving the Wall Street world represented a serious correction.

On the advice of Bob Albo, Geoff decided to adopt a halfway measure; he would keep his post and commute between Hong Kong and San Francisco. It would be a demanding travel schedule. Every 20 days Geoff would fly to California to spend the chemotherapy period with me, including the overnight stays in the hospital. He would return to Hong Kong the following week. It was the best solution we could come up with. Not only could I not imagine Geoff having to leave his work completely while I was under treatment, but there was another aspect. Had the doctors told Geoff to quit his job, I would have suspected them of hiding a dark prognosis.

There was also the question of where I would stay while going through treatment. And what about our youngest child, Caroline, who had already started school in Hong Kong? I felt that her place was with me. I began asking for help with the smallest questions in my prayers, and once the chemotherapy regime began, these considerations seemed to resolve themselves.

Cindy and her husband had built their dream house in Marin County just a year before. Included in the plan was a small, one room cottage called, "Whippet," which my wonderful brother-in-law completed for me within six weeks of the lymphoma diagnosis. The name of the cottage was an excellent reminder of what I had to do. It was decided that I would stay there during the chemotherapy treatments. It was cozy and very comfortable, private but nearby, in case I needed help. We had heard stories of body temperatures plummeting at night, and other complications related to chemotherapy. Not knowing what was to come, I was enormously relieved not to be alone.

"Whippet," named before I came, was an idyllic little dream. In full sunlight or in early morning fog, it is a warm and beckoning place. I was near my sister, who, through this illness, became my dearest friend.

We solved the schooling question and overrode the wishes of a formidably stern Scottish headmistress in Hong Kong, who had wanted to advance Caroline to the next grade. Six weeks into term, the private school in Marin County was full, with the exception of one place in The Lower School. The vacancy was in our daughter's grade. Caroline was welcomed and beautifully looked after there. The school had a loving atmosphere and was academically challenging. It also had horses, her main passion in life. Caroline could ride twice a week. It was another perfect solution in a chain of beautifully placed "coincidences."

I approached the chemotherapy sessions in a positive way. I had a room with a view, which was pleasing, and a fine team of nurses, many of whom became friends. There were always flowers on the bedside table and a loving husband who stayed with me. Sometimes that meant sleeping on a mat on the floor.

On Bernie Siegel's advice I learned to bless the difficult treatments. The chemicals were not the enemy, but the helpers. It was not easy, but it was possible to be thankful. The chemotherapy regime and the doctor who oversaw it bought me invaluable time in which to jump-start the fuller healing process: the healing of a life—mind, body and spirit.

When my hair began to fall out, determined not to feel like a victim, I cut it off. By Christmas, when it had become scraggly and sporadic in length, I covered my head with shaving foam and shaved it clean. Hesitating to look in the mirror at Telly Savalas, there was a nice surprise. I had never seen my eyes in such an isolated setting before; they looked surprisingly wonderful.

I was conscious of having moved into Bernie Siegel's Exceptional Cancer Patient's Club. Although physically weakened and tired by the treatments, I knew I would not be a statistic. I went on to tell myself that I was getting well. In and out of fear, brave and not brave, and with the humility that can only accompany an uncharted course, I kept coming back to it. With help from my angels, to whom I spoke daily and had begun to know, I would get well. I would listen, evaluate, and trust the leaps of faith. Anyway, this was my best plan.

One of the nurses confided that in the second month of treatment, my hospital file was marked on the outside with capital letters: "EXCEPTIONAL PATIENT." Bernie Siegel is good.

6

Truth has many faces and the truth is like to the old road to Avalon; it depends on your own will and your own thoughts whither the road will take you.

—Marion Zimmer-Bradley,
author of *The Mists of Avalon*

As far as I can remember it was mid-October when the pennies first started to appear. The first one I found was miles from home in the parking lot of a large shopping mall. Cindy drove into a parking space, and as I stepped out of the car, it was there on the pavement.

"How nice," I thought, "a shining little piece of luck."

I picked it up, smiled, and put it into my pocket.

"Every little bit helps," we laughed.

Two days later there would be another and then another. They appeared in any number of places: in a friend's driveway, at the library, in a store, a restaurant, or at the Ladies Room at the San Francisco Airport. They appeared all over creation. After two months I counted them and worked out the frequency with which they appeared. I was finding a penny approximately every three days.

This number held for about six months, as long as the chemotherapy treatments lasted. Funnily enough, after that they tapered off. When the pennies were flowing, I found doubles on some days. If four days passed without finding one, I would begin watching for them, but under those circumstances they would never appear. Once, on a morning walk, I paused to shake a pebble out of my shoe. Stooping down to put it back on, I saw a penny there, on the dirt pathway. "Thank you." I would pick each one up, salute it, and put it with the others in the side pocket of the car door. Soon the pocket had a definite bulge.

For a while, the magical appearance of these pennies seemed lightly amusing. Over time they became a sort of presence. Cindy and I told Geoff about them and asked what he thought.

"We have lived outside of America during a time that the currency has devalued considerably," he said. "The penny isn't worth anything anymore. People probably just throw them away." It seemed a logical explanation. We shrugged our shoulders and felt a little silly for having asked.

But a month later he expanded his evaluation.

"The strange thing is that the pennies seem to find you. They never find Cindy or me. I agree with you; it's peculiar."

Soon the pennies moved me to another dimension in which I felt blessed. This feeling would softly wrap itself around me and tears would follow. It was as though someone was putting a loving arm around me. The pennies let me know that I was not alone. Something or someone was very near, somehow looking after me. But who, or what could it be?

For several years, as a summertime hobby I had read a great deal about the American Indians. Could these spirits be nearby? The philosophy of Chief Seattle had become mine.

"How can you buy the sky? How can you own the rain and the wind?...The voice of my grandfather said to me, the air is precious. It shares its spirit with all the life it supports. The wind that gave me my first breath also received my last sigh. You must keep the land and air apart and sacred, as a place where one can go to taste the wind that is sweetened by the meadow flowers."

Native ceremonies and music were captivating, and although an outsider, I felt a certain quiet, unassuming kinship with them. At one point just before we learned that I was ill, a hummingbird followed me for fifteen minutes, hovering closely near my left arm as Caroline and I walked in our Tahoe woods. We marveled at this creature. The experience left us both feeling complimented somehow. A friend told me later that animals and children only come to you if you have a good and loving aura. I hoped this was so.

Black Elk, a Lakota Indian Shaman, describes animal behavior during sacred ceremonies. He tells of the gathering of forest animals, of foxes sitting next to rabbits, and other natural enemies coming together peacefully in a circle while the shaman commemorates their relationship to the whole of nature.

I had also collected jewelry made by the Navajo, the Hopi and the Zuni Indians. There was one particular fetish necklace, a great favorite, which I wore to the hospital every treatment time: the fox, the bear, the eagle, and turtle all went around my neck. They were friends, and there was a measure of security and comfort in traveling with this crowd.

Perhaps because of this interest in Indian lore, a very dear friend in New York City told me about an intriguing and eloquent Hungarian-born anthropologist, Dr. Felicitas Goodman. Dr. Goodman is head of The Cuyamungue Institute near Santa Fe in New Mexico. In her book, *Where the Spirits Ride the Wind*, she describes a spiritual encounter she had in New Mexico.

On her way to a Memorial Mass for an old Indian, called Tom, Dr. Goodman felt that something representing the Indian spirit should be included at the altar.

"I was alone, so I said out loud, 'Please, my Friend, do come along to comfort the spirit of Old Tom. Attach yourself to my left shoulder and be my companion.' Being new to the path of the Spirits, I was thoroughly shaken when there was an instantaneous response. Coming up from behind, a tremendous ball of force hit me squarely on the left side of my body. But bewilderment soon gave way to a sense of companionship and a delicious feeling of conspiracy, which stayed with me as I walked into the valley down the hot and dusty trail."

Dr. Goodman's book made me wonder about the pennies. For a time I thought a playful Indian spirit might have put them in my pathway. Many stories describe Indian spirits as having a great sense of humor. I put these suspicions to one side, hoping in time to understand.

Late in November Cindy and her business partner arranged for me to go with them to meet Lawrence Stoller, who was at that time called The Crystal Master of Northern California. Neither Cindy nor I knew anything at all about crystals, but the "power of coincidence" came into play. Cindy's business partner had recently sold Lawrence and his wife, Sunni, their house in Mill Valley, a charming city located in the woods of Marin County.

The house was well-sited, tucked into a wooded hillside with enormous spreading oak trees, dappled shade, and on this clear day, a squeegee-clear blue sky above. The house was a giant adult treehouse with vast expanses of glass. The day was planned as an instructive and enjoyable outing, but the chemotherapy treatments had been exhausting. While the oncologist had classified me as "doing well," I tired easily and spent a lot of energy trying to disguise the fact that my spirit and feet were dragging.

We spent the better part of an autumn afternoon with Lawrence. He and his pigeon-toed Sun Conyer provided a walking tour of the mineral kingdom and the cutting workshop. There were boxes of rocks from all over the world to be cut, polished and shipped for sale. The finished ones were majestic casings for rainbows and images of all sorts, which could be discovered by holding them up to the sun's light.

One large yellow crystal was displayed in the living room, standing over two feet tall, with an even wider girth. Lawrence took great joy in his work. He explained that gems and crystals have been treasured and worn as talismans for thousands of years. One thinks of the Chinese valuing jade, the American Indians and the Tibetans, turquoise, and the Incas, emeralds. Royal families have always adorned themselves with crowns of diamonds, rubies, and a myriad of other precious stones.

Crystals have been used in specific ways since prehistoric times. Interacting with light, they produce an energy, which neutralizes negative vibrations and heightens consciousness. This happens whether one is aware of the crystals as having power or not.

The colors of the gems correspond to the colors of our main chakras, or energy centers. From the base chakra at the bottom of the spine to the crown chakra above the head, the color order is red/black, red/orange, orange/yellow, green or pink/blue, indigo/violet, and gold or white. Each chakra is believed to be physiological as well as spiritual in nature.

Rose quartz, for example would normally be used to restore or calm the heart chakra. The energy which it generates relates to inner peace and self-fulfillment. It is a comforting stone, soothing to the troubled or broken heart.

Amethyst, the purple mineral, is connected to spiritual growth, and is often placed on the lower half of the forehead, over the Third Eye. At one time in the history of man, the amethyst was valued at parity with diamonds. It was the gem representing the Inner World, or the spirit; the diamond denoted the Outer World, the commercial and materialistic realm. Noting the modern day appreciation of these gems, it is easy to deduce the direction in which the world has evolved.

Lawrence cuts healing crystals for medical doctors, who use them in a complimentary way in their traditional medical practices. It was one of these crystals that I ultimately bought, a beautiful piece of quartz from Madagascar, with traces of sparkling pyrite inside. Of all the crystals in the collection, this was the one I was drawn to: for its shape, color and for the silvery flakes inside, which seemed to me to be significant.

Lawrence taught me how to cleanse and clear the crystal by soaking it in water overnight. Weeks later I learned how to program each facet for healing. Because of the asymmetrical way in which the crystal was cut, I could identify individual facets in the dark, simply by feeling them.

Lawrence, with his elfin grin and sparkling blue eyes added, "Some people actually talk to their crystals, you know, they do!"

I paid him for the crystal and put it in my handbag. When we were putting our jackets on, he asked me, almost casually, if I knew why I got sick.

"What do you mean?"

"Do you know what is at the bottom of the illness?"

"No, I can't tell you. I don't know. I don't really know what you mean."

"Where was the cancer?" Lawrence asked.

"In the abdominal area."

"In the solar plexus," he filled in, and then paused. "It is probably old anger," he said, "accumulated anger and hurt."

"Really? I'll think about what you are saying, but I honestly don't think I have any anger at all!"

In gentleness he did not say, That's the worst variety, the deeply buried and hidden kind.

Instead, he said, "Look and see. You need to find out."

"I guess I do."

"You must," he said firmly, "or you will get sick again. Do you want help?"

"I suppose so." I said.

"Have you ever heard of Lazaris?"

"I learned of him in Hong Kong. He is the spiritual entity who speaks through Jack Purcell." This time I was smiling to myself and thought, Who arranged all of this?

"Lazaris is the best. Get his audiotape, *On Releasing Anger*, as soon as you can. He will help you get started. You can also write to him and ask for a telephone consultation. The waiting list is long, but you can probably work something out."

"How long is it?"

"Usually about three years; but he keeps time slots open for people with health emergencies. He will probably talk to you right away. Just explain what you are going through. But listen to his tape first and see what you think."

When we got to the car, he moved further into the drive and called after us, "One more thing," he said, racing to catch up, "there aren't any coincidences, you know, just surprises." Then he stopped, smiled and waved us off.

We ran into a New Age Bookstore in Mill Valley and bought the Lazaris tape, *On Releasing Anger*, and listened to it on the way home.

7

No man is your friend; no man is your enemy; every man is your teacher.

—Anonymous

Most of us know that there is a relationship between the general health of the body and the health of the mind and spirit. We may have read about stress hormones, which have been shown to contribute to chronic depression. Fast-paced lives with little or no attention to balance are known to shorten our years. Norman Cousins wrote about the healing power of humor, extending his life, as he laughed his way through two serious illnesses. With an introduction to the Lazaris material, I began to see that the mind-body relationship is profoundly basic, increasingly obvious.

I began to shift my mind in new directions, analyzing the old assumptions, which had served in my life as the silent, insidious dictators.

In Western societies we are taught to please our families and to fit into the group. As a side effect we learn to bury anger, resentment and authenticity, among other things. It is not considered attractive, especially for girls, to speak out or to raise their voices. We learn to put our needs aside, and to hide hurt feelings as not to look weak or wimpy, in need of attention. There is a link between people pleasing and what we learn about acceptability and love.

Everyone knows that most of what we know about love we learn from our parents or primary care givers very early in life. Can we trust other human beings? Are we deserving of love and regard? We stay within this maternal and paternal definition throughout life unless a conscious choice is made to examine and to redefine it all for ourselves.

Love in the family in which I was a child, was supportive in most ways and fiercely loyal. It was also about being considerate and thoughtful, with mind reading on the part of the children expected. It was not the kind of love that held you close or let you feel how special you were. Nor did it rock you to sleep.

I don't believe that this was unusual. My sense from reading, listening to interviews and speaking to other War Babies is that this was fairly normal within American families in the 1940s and 1950s. It was a time for hard work as the working class sensed tremendous post-war opportunity and seized it, hoping to capture The Good Life.

Without thinking, I demonstrated the kind of love I was familiar with, blindly and without question, supporting my husband's Wall Street career and our children's development. This is what I was supposed to do. It was my job. It didn't seem difficult, and I was extremely strong. Everyone counted on that. If I had any needs, I believed they could wait for a more convenient time. I would get to them later. It was in the open-ended waiting that my life became inauthentic. Still, I was just doing my job, as women have done for centuries. Many of my friends had husbands with high-powered careers; I did comparison checks, and determined that our lives were quite similar. We were all ambitious, sensible, and self-sacrificing, in pursuit of an even better Good Life. But for me the price of admission was high.

It was time to review old beliefs and perspectives, then to test their source and validity. Is this attitude a helpful one, or is it limiting? Is it promoting good health? If the old patterns were removed or altered, would I somehow melt away? Putting it another way, don't our belief systems figuratively hold us together? In changing mine, would I become someone I didn't know or like? This aspect of the healing process was as formidable as the challenge presented by the cancer, itself.

The first belief questioned was: Why is it necessary to hide and bury nearly all of my emotions? Answer: Because I have always thought of myself as a very strong person, a linchpin for family, friends and associates, and this is what strong people do. This is how they behave. It is necessary. But why does this seem to be so? The invaluable answer came in a quiet meditative time, in a memory as clear as clear, as if it had been recorded on film.

I was in second grade; it was just after Easter. We had a substitute teacher on that day, and I had brought a large sugar shell egg to show my classmates. It was decorated with squiggles of hard yellow frosting and had a scene inside. If you held it up to one eye, there was a magical family of rabbits inside working in their flower garden. This egg was something special. Father Rabbit pushed a wheelbarrow and wore a tie. In the course of Share and Tell, the teacher asked if I would mind passing the egg around the class. I took an undetectably deep breath and said that it would be OK.

My friend, Lawrence, sat on the far left of the classroom, second seat from the front. He was a very nice boy, with jet-black curly hair, who wore white, crisply ironed shirts. When the egg was passed on to him, he dropped it and it shattered. Collectively there was an air-sucking gasp. After a few moments I went over to him and told him not to feel bad, and meant it. We swept the sugar pieces into a dustpan. He was very sorry and embarrassed.

At the end of the day, Mother came to school to walk me home, visiting first with the substitute teacher. Already anticipating some sort of tearful scene on the way home, I overheard the teacher complimenting her on how grown-up I was, how "advanced for my age."

"Lynne is going to be a very strong leader," she said. "I can see that in just one day. She didn't cry or make a fuss at all when her special Easter egg was broken. She is a remarkable child."

Mother was thrilled and very proud of me, as any mother would have been. In the chemistry of that moment I was seduced by the compliment and buried any thoughts of crying. Strong people don't do it. None of us understood the dynamics which were established that day, but within moments I had assimilated the teacher's compliment and her definitions of strength and leadership, and grafted them onto the center of my small first grade self. For all the tears I would never shed and feelings denied expression, under the guise of strength and leadership I was on the way to trouble.

Feelings are manifested in the body; if stressful emotions are held in, they do us great harm. I never knew about this when I was growing up. I don't believe many people did. Lazaris was the first one to come along and explain this to me.

One of the many reasons I came to admire Lazaris is that he emphasizes individual responsibility. It is incumbent upon each of us to listen carefully to divine inner guidance, and then to choose among the choices, which are presented to us. After choosing, we act, we evaluate, and then we listen again. In this process of reflection we can grow and begin to heal our lives.

Lazaris was placed in my path in Hong Kong and once more in America. By the time I really needed him as a teacher and friend, his unusual abilities were more familiar, and my resistance softened.

While Cindy and I listened to his audiotape, *On Releasing Anger*, Lazaris had a stunning message. He teaches that in and of itself, anger is not a negative emotion. It can, in fact, be quite positive. I quite agree; but there is a catch.

"*Suppressed* anger is lethal," he explains. "You honestly cannot afford to delay unlocking and releasing it. Unlike other debilitating forces it does not lie dormant within you until you are ready to work with it. It is actively destroying you."

Anger is a liberating force when it is spent or expended. Lazaris suggests beginning by writing a letter to someone whom has made you angry:

> Dear _____,
>
> Moving through the healing process, I realize that there are a lot of things I need to talk to you about so that I can be freed of them. We have developed patterns in our relationship which have hurt me, and I want to change them. Without wanting or meaning to I have harbored negative feelings, which have contributed to making our relationship worse and to making me sick. They have to do with how you have treated me and my children. I know that you have played sinisterly clever games with us in the past for reasons I don't understand.
>
> I will telephone you after you receive this to see if we can get together to talk soon. Next Tuesday or Wednesday would be a good time for me.
>
> More later,

Depending on the outcome of this initial step, time with this other person is arranged. If the first step is futile, or if the individual involved is not receptive, what would be a forced meeting need not take place. In the process of trying to release anger it is, after all, counterproductive to set yourself up for accumulating more. The challenge in this kind of situation is to unilaterally, genuinely forgive the individual who caused you pain, to transform it with understanding and compassion, and to forgive yourself for allowing it to happen. Then it is possible to let them go on their way (whether a part of your life or not), wishing them well. The process can be quite long and arduous; it can be quick. In any case it is crucial.

Lazaris describes the value and the precise technique of the Hate Letter. This type of letter is written, edited and rewritten in a prescribed way, four or five times within a certain time frame. Sometimes the letter is actually posted; more often it is burned. One of mine took 20 minutes to burn on the barbecue in Hong Kong.

> Dear _____,
>
> It is so unbelievable to me that when I was a little girl you used to pester my mother for me to come and stay with you. Once she would drop me off you completely ignored me! And you were mean. Why? What kind of creepy, deprived person are you to deliberately hurt a small child like that! You were sinister and malicious, an abusive, horrible person. I think you are a psychopathic personality and I really don't want to be around you. I don't know why I ever had to have you in my life.
>
> And sign it in an inspired way.

As Lazaris explains, it is possible to have many different layers of anger, going back to childhood. If you were five years old (or twelve or twenty-three), it is very important to recapture the emotion as you felt it then. It can be exploded with the release of tears by punching pillows, screaming, whatever is effective. (It is best to follow the procedure as described on Lazaris' tape.)

Lazaris goes on to explain that most major health problems are products of repressed anger.

"The most catastrophic anger [is that] of cancer," he says, "[an] anger so deeply and totally repressed that many times people don't honestly know they have it. It may take ten years, maybe twenty years, but the anger will be processed through a self-destructive cancer that will eat away and totally destroy the body."

Lazaris helped me begin to undo the catastrophic state I found myself in by teaching me to find my feelings and honor them.

Another excellent teacher during this period of discovery was Dr. O. Carl Simonton. A pioneering oncologist, Dr. Simonton describes in great detail the emotions which cause serious problems. On his audiotape, *Getting Well*, and in his book, *Stress, Psychological Factors and Cancer*, he speaks of "core beliefs." Is the world a positive or a negative dog-eat-dog place? Is everyone out to get me? To swindle or take advantage of me? Are people basically good or evil? These beliefs can be insidiously hidden and negative. Conversely, if we believe that Mankind is basically good, this will be a positive influence. Childhood beliefs are passed on from one generation to the next in what I think of as cultural genetics.

Dr. Simonton goes on to demonstrate how we can slowly change the parts of our personality which put us at risk, and thereby learn to deal more happily and effectively with daily life.

At this point I also became acquainted with Louise Hay's work and began to use positive affirmations in the healing process. When a critical remark would enter my mind, I noticed it and let it go by, immediately affirming, "I release the need to be hypercritical and judgmental, to always have an opinion." If I became cross over something I might have done poorly or left undone, "I love and approve of myself exactly as I am." Worrying about the cancer, "I am open to receive and maintain perfect health." Affirmations are splendid, powerful tools, which can be life altering.

Someone very dear to me once said, "How can I look in the mirror and say, 'I love and approve of myself' when I don't? In fact I think I am disgusting and I don't believe in affirmations anyway."

"You have just made one, and it isn't one that is going to help you. Can you start by saying, 'I am open now to learning how to love and approve of myself?" I asked.

Thinking of the role that personality has to play, as children, my sister and I had two very different reactions to the same recurring event. It was quite significant in my life and not at all important in hers.

When Cindy and I were young, Mother had heart attacks with some frequency. She had a leaking heart valve, the result of having contracted rheumatic fever as a child. Holding fast to her religious beliefs, she refused medical treatment. Mother believed that, as a Christian Scientist, she could demonstrate perfect healing through prayer. Three or four times a year she would collapse on the forest green sofa in the living room and stay there for an hour or more, with her eyes closed, heart thumping. (Twenty years later Mother's extremely erratic heartbeat was described by a heart specialist as "the most incredible EKG I have ever seen.")

Being the responsible and conscientious older child, I tried to help, and as there was no one else around, I took charge in my own way. I was eight years old when I first became aware of the attacks. Each time it happened I thought my Mother was going to die.

Mommy might not get up this time, I remember thinking. This could be the end.

I can remember covering her with a cozy lap robe, getting a blanket for myself, and sliding down the side of the sofa onto the floor, just sitting there with my chin on my knees.

"Oh please, God, don't let her die this time, not this time."

She didn't die, and as time went by I came to believe that she would be fine as long as I held the vigil. After a while, the fear moved into a new and ironically practical direction. Numbed by a series of these experiences, I began to project worries into the future. I didn't know how to cook. What would I do if Mother never got up from the green sofa again? Someone would have to prepare dinner. It would have to be me. Daddy is pretty hopeless. All he can cook are Swedish pancakes. They wouldn't be suitable. I could probably figure out macaroni and cheese and a salad, but would it turn out well?

A peculiar aspect of this memory is that I never cried; nor did I feel that I could intervene in the adults' world and mention this, not even to my special grandmother. It seems particularly odd that my mother and I never talked about it. And so the episodes remained a secret. All I could do was to keep the vigil at my mother's side and pray and hope. Inside I was petrified, but no one ever knew. I willed my mother to live, and as far as I could tell, it worked.

Cindy, on the other hand, was the second born, known as Scarlett O'Hara for her sense of "Fiddle-de-dee. I'll think about it tomorrow." She would peer around the corner of the living room, see Mother on the sofa, me on the floor, and run out the door to play.

After I got sick and came to understand how devastating this childhood memory was for me, I asked Cindy with some annoyance whatever she thought during those times. Why was I all alone trying to save our Mother? Why did I have to be the responsible one?

"How could you just run outside?" I asked her.

"I thought, 'Oh! Mom's on the sofa again. It's something she does every now and then.' I didn't think it was important. It meant that I could play outside longer with my friends."

Two children, three and a half years apart in age, same family, same environment, and two very different responses, a testimony to two very distinct personalities and roles. The irony was that of the two of us my sister grew up to be the more compassionate one. She felt deep concern for people and for animals. Often bringing stray dogs home, she would telephone their owners and arrange for them to be picked up. When she was old enough to drive she would rescue two or three dogs from pound executions and find homes for them. She was by far more demonstrative and affectionate than I was. Of course our personalities were different, but compassion was something that I now believe I had shut down, as I sat beside the green sofa. It came out of dormancy and magically changed my life when I became ill.

Between my parents, Mother's heart attacks were barely an issue. My father, who is an intelligent and accepting man, respected her religious beliefs and wishes. Mother is a strong Nordic woman, who tends to hold the dominant point of view. But I was the one who was affected profoundly. Coupled with fear and anxiety, there was the latent element of anger. ("Who is in charge here? I don't want to be in charge. I want to be the child.") I grew to believe that no one in my family paid attention to significant details but me.

I took on the job of the "responsible human being," always focused on the task at hand and the needs of others. Personalities are hewn this way. We bend and fit, turn and match. Women, especially, are taught to please, to help and support, and to become players in what often becomes a whole slew of co-dependent relationships. Now a mature adult, I was molded to be the perfect spouse for a demanding workaholic. I always coped, supported, and kept the vigil for the others. It was now time for me to do this for myself.

8

It is only with the heart that one can see rightly; what is essential is invisible to the eye.

—*The Little Prince*, by Antoine de Saint-Exupery

As the chemotherapy treatments continued I supposed that I was doing very well. At the same time, having never been through this kind of experience before, there was no way of knowing what doing well meant. My only physical complaint was that I tired extremely easily and my stomach was upset following meals. The lab reports showed that my body was holding up to a rigorous regimen of chemicals and steroids, but at this point no one in the medical world knew how effective the six month treatment would be.

While the doctors waited, I felt I had nothing to lose and possibly a lifetime to gain by investigating alternative approaches. I set aside quiet time to rest and to give myself Reiki Treatments every day, with either Lazaris or the Simonton tapes playing on the Walkman. It was in this period that something very unusual happened.

Fear was, as always, an obstreperous, nasty wild card. From the beginning I likened it to The Hook in the old vaudevillian shows I had seen something about on television. It would appear out of nowhere and grab you by the neck, on a perfectly nice day, in a wonderful place, at an innocent moment. It would sneak up on me, and cling tenaciously, pulling me down and down and down to a horrible place of paranoia and helplessness. Hopes were shattered, progress dishonored and faith in the miracles so far, rendered to be utter nonsense. It was silly, and I was deceiving myself. Why did I think I was going to survive following these "other" methods? The unconventional track I had chosen was just another form of denial. At times like these it seemed that everyone around me felt this way. In 1989 I felt myself to be a lone explorer who had chosen to follow some very bizarre directions. The truth seemed to be that this was all a foolish and very risky exercise. And where was the methodology, anyway? Following angels or instincts? How foolhardy! How irresponsible! What a dope! As if on cue, a phantom chorus of medical doctors would put in their two cents: "Forget all of this and get yourself to Stanford Medical School to be evaluated for a bone marrow transplant. After all, you know what your prognosis is. Here are the numbers and the graphs. These are your odds." The demons would temporarily convince me that faith, belief, hope and healing were all figments of an exceedingly desperate imagination.

But then, after a few hours, sometimes a few days, I would emerge from this doomsday place, climb out of the black hole back to the well-lighted healing place which fear had tried so hard to obliterate.

It is an irony how we simply forget the miracles which have helped us to move forward. I had the pennies, the help of a presence which I called "my angels," and the support of family and friends. I was, after all, doing well. Once all of these pieces were put back into place, I could climb up again. In allowing myself to feel the blessings, there was a freedom and hopefulness once more. I would dust myself off and begin again, ready to move on to more of the positives.

In the beginning the angels were without faces. They did not appear as figures with wings in gauze dresses. Yet they seemed to be impeccably organized. I felt them to be a group, but wasn't sure I had given them the right name. They were invisible forces of loving kindness and mysterious support, and I knew they were near me a good deal of the time.

One evening in December I went out to Whippet for a rest. As I had recently had a chemotherapy treatment, Geoff was still in California. He was sitting at the kitchen table in the Big House preparing to call the office. On the other side of the world, Hong Kong was just waking up.

It was after five o'clock, darkness had begun to settle in, and the sky looked like the auditorium of a planetarium. It was a bowl-shaped silhouette with eucalyptus and crisp evergreen forms all around. Venus, the Evening Star, shone brilliantly noble in the heavens. Someone in the neighborhood had a fire burning, adding a softly beckoning element to the crisp night air on the walk between the Big House and Whippet.

Once in the cottage, I tucked in under the duvet, which would soon be snuggly and warm, reached for the healing crystal, and turned out the light.

No tapes this time, I thought. I would just hold the crystal and give myself a Reiki treatment, following the same process which Nancy

Beckor had used, but with my own hands. Sinking into the coziness of the goose down, I closed my eyes and began to relax.

Lawrence Stoller came into my thoughts. How glad I was to have met him and to have the crystal. It fit my hand perfectly and had become a sort of friend, lovely to look at, pleasant to hold. But the part which made me smile even more that evening was the bizarre notion that people speak to their crystals. My Swedish grandmother would have said, "The crazy don't have it all alike." Then she would have laughed, including herself among them.

To my great surprise, in less than a minute, I heard my own voice, though the words seemed to be spoken by someone else. Was this a self-imposed impish joke? Completely unplanned, I heard myself speaking to the crystal. Moving my right thumb on the facet programmed for perfect health and long life, I said, "I want to be completely healthy and to live a long and wonderful life."

From behind closed eyes, colors flashed on my mental screen, much as they had during the Reiki treatments in Hong Kong. But this time there was a more vibrant periwinkle blue, thrown like a bucket of Disney cartoon paint. The splash was curly around the edges with a few maverick drops around the periphery. It was astonishing.

"How beautiful!" I said. "I don't know what this is, but thank you."

Another color appeared. From the center of the blue splash came a vibrant magenta-pink. It was glowing, as though an incandescent light were shining behind it. The light was warm and mellow.

I watched for some time as the magenta came and went. I can't be sure for how long, but it carried me away. Not only were the colors phenomenal, but the timing!

When it was over, my mental screen simply went dark again, and I was dropped back into the ordinary night in the regular world. I sat up in bed, still holding the crystal, and cried. Sitting in the darkness with tears running down my face, I accepted this vividly reassuring response with a sense of awe and blessing. Whatever was going on was comforting and, like the pennies, made me feel much less alone.

The Hook lost much of its power after that. It still could pull me down to the depths, to the same doomsday place, but with far less regularity.

Afterward I tried to rest, but couldn't. I went into the Big House. Geoff was all alone, still working at the table in the kitchen. I told him what had happened. Poor man. I can't imagine what he thought. He didn't know what to make of it, but he could tell it was important. He locked me in his arms and held on.

I wondered: would I have seen the colors if I had spoken without the crystals in my hand? Who could say? I am very sure that when we ask with sincerity for something we are heard. And if we are open and clear enough to receive help, we are supported, often in mysterious ways.

Weeks later my father said, "I don't know how we explain these things, but I do know that the experience you had dissolved most of your fear. It was a gift, you know. You were a different person after that. You started to relax. That is a miracle, isn't it?"

The next morning I awakened thinking about a book found some weeks before, by a British Reverend, Theo Gimbel, called *Healing through Color*. Because of an interest in design and textiles, I had bought a copy. Upon opening it I wondered if it might be a sort of codebook. I looked up the two colors I had been shown the night before to see if there was any reference to their significance or meaning. (pg. 151)

> *BLUE*: of all the colours this [is] the most healing... It is the light of peace, relaxing the whole body, regulating the harmonious development of tissue.
>
> *MAGENTA*: this colour draws man into spiritual awareness. It can be used only rarely, and it would be good to keep this colour for the special purposes of transmitting from the denser realms into the spiritual field; a color more for the mature person.

Fascinating. I thumbed through other pages with the enthusiasm of a gold miner about to strike pay dirt. On page 63 another light bulb went on. A small chart related colors to different parts of the body:

> *YELLOW*: represents the solar plexus/stomach

The two fried eggs zoomed into focus. The C-T Scan had indicated only one lymphoma tumor, but, in fact, Bob Albo found what he described as two lemon-shaped tumors in the solar plexus area. It seemed incredible. What were the pussy willows then? This was more difficult. Eventually it was clear that they represented liver involvement. The fact that they had appeared on a periwinkle ground was reassuring.

It was a genuine "Aha!" experience.

But moments later, in typically human fashion, it seemed too far-fetched. How can one read an experience like this? Last year I didn't know where the blooming solar plexus was, and now I was hooking it up with crazy colored charts.

Now here were the interpretations. The problem was that they came from a realm which I didn't know well and was hard-pressed to trust.

Could this illness be the voyage I had been so anxious to get on with? More tears. It was too scary. I didn't want to take this journey anymore. Cancel the trip.

9

God created man because he loves stories.

—Isaak Dinesen

In meditation I found strength and comfort in images from my childhood. Over a period of a week, the images connected and became a continuous stream. They were all of Nana, my Swedish Grandmother. The scenes always began in the same way. I would be sitting at her kitchen table with a cup of hot cocoa, dangling my long and lanky legs, blowing on the cup and enjoying our time together.

"Will you tell me one of the stories about India?" I would ask. She had related them hundreds of times, but the stories were never boring. They were a living part of my family's history. And then, they were magic carpets, a guaranteed ride to exotic adventures. It wasn't until I was an adult with children of my own that I smiled one day with the realization that Nana had felt the same.

"Which story would you like to hear?" she would say. "You know them all."

"Tell me about the magpie who stole the first mate's wife's diamond ring off the window sill while she washed her hands at The Great Eastern Hotel in Calcutta." Then I would change my mind, close my eyes and choose another. "No, tell me the one about the python that bit the Indian lady on her bottom."

My eyes would widen, and forgetting about the hot chocolate, I would spread my elbows flat onto the table, rest my face on my hands, and become quiet.

"Well," Nana began, "a conscientious old snake keeper in New Delhi was worried about one of his friends, who happened to be a python. These snakes are very common in India. They swallow animals whole, you remember."

"Tell me again what they swallow."

"They eat rats and mice, rabbits, birds even small goats, all sorts of small creatures. They help to maintain the balance of nature. One dark night your grandfather had to bicycle through the jungle in Ceylon. He hit a big bump on the path and almost fell over. The next day he went back and discovered that he had run over a python with what must have been a baby goat in its belly."

How delightfully disgusting it was.

"How scary to be on a bicycle in a dark jungle."

"But we have to get back to the snake keeper in New Delhi. It was the weekend, you see, the time when the old man was scheduled to have his day off, but the snake, who lived at the zoo, was feeling poorly. The keeper, who was a kind-hearted man, decided to take the snake home and put it in the bathroom in his small flat. It seemed like a sensible idea. In this way the man could have a weekend without worrying about the snake and the snake would be well looked after.

"Having spent a very easy night, the old keeper checked his friend the following morning and quickly saw that the recuperative regime was working. The snake was much better. He decided to go out and get some live food for him.

"The old man closed the bathroom door, latched it, and off he went to the bazaar. About one hour later he returned to find hysterical women everywhere, running around with their hands held to their ears, elbows up to the sky, their shiny black braids bobbing on their backs. They were panicked. The python was loose! The python was loose! Oh dear.

"The snake keeper hadn't thought about the latrine as a place where a snake might have an adventure, but he soon figured it out. The snake had gone down the old man's toilet and come up in someone else's, a large Indian woman's, as she was having a private time in her bathroom."

For a young child this part was absolutely delicious.

"The woman claimed she was bitten on the backside and was in plenty of pain, but the newspaper said that she wouldn't let anyone examine her.

"Eventually the old man calmed everyone down, found the snake, fed him a few very delicious mice (who had nearly escaped themselves), and took the python back to the zoo."

It was a good story. It still is. They were all like that. Nana and I had always been kindred spirits; the stories enhanced our connection and set us apart. There was so much to learn from her. She was a well-traveled person, quite brave and a character in her own right. Although she wasn't cuddly (Swedes aren't known to be), I drew the greatest emotional sustenance from her. She was my biggest hero, and I adored her.

When my father was a little boy of four, she and my grandfather took him on a trip with them. They sailed around the world for a couple of years. My Danish grandfather was the ship's captain. In 1918 they all nearly perished just outside the port of Trincomalee, off the coast of Ceylon.

"It had rained and blown for nearly seven days, and it was clear that the motorship, *City of St. Helens*, was going to go down. What do you think you would take with you if you had to abandon ship? I don't know why, but along with clean underwear for the three of us, I packed the movie camera and the film. Then I began to worry about the monkey onboard who didn't have a tail. He was handicapped and would need help, but I couldn't find him anywhere. In the end the joke was on me, because he had been hiding for days under the tarp inside one of the lifeboats. Clever little fellow!"

I loved the monkey.

"The storm finally cleared, the miracle we had all prayed for. The floorboards in the engine room were barely intact, and the sails were shredded to ribbons. It took six months in the boatyard to restore her. Lloyds of London sent a beautiful black car for us, and your Daddy and I were driven to Kandy, in the hills, so that we could stay in a place where it was cool, while your grandfather went to Colombo to oversee repairs."

Nana adored Ceylon. She could never bring herself to call it by its modern name. She told me once that her most cherished memories were there, possibly because life felt especially sweet when the certainty of immediate death was removed. It is like that in the calming reprieve after a horrific monsoon.

Ceylon is an unusually lush and beautiful island. Nana and my father used to go down to the river to see the elephants have their bath. They were scrubbed with big stiff brushes.

"If the elephants didn't have their baths every day, they would lie down on the ground and refuse to work. It was as though they went on strike," Nana would say. "Aren't they intelligent creatures?"

My grandfather was a fine and capable but stern man. He was a Dane and a strict disciplinarian. He never drank and he disliked foul language, which must have been a surprise to his seafaring crews. On land he ate fruit all of the time, I remember. I supposed it was because he couldn't get enough fresh food at sea. I also remember that he was forever trying to give Nana orders. She would listen and nod, then do as she pleased.

He called her "My Little Honey Dear." She was beautiful and he adored her.

The day they arrived in Port Said, he instructed Nana to stay onboard while he went ashore to see the Freight Agents. Once he was out of sight, Nana convinced the first mate, a jolly Dane and loyal friend, called Uncle Charlie, to row her ashore with my father, who was only four, so they could have ice cream.

"We were sitting in a small cafe, Uncle Charlie and your daddy and I, talking and laughing. It was so good to be on land again. When who do you think came riding by in a rickshaw grand as you please, sitting tall under his toupee, but your grandfather. He looked very handsome. We hid behind the menus, laughing and whispering, but the menus were small and flimsy, so as he came nearer we slid down in our chairs. Your daddy thought it was lots of fun! So did I. It was a perfect crime."

Nana's stories were enchanting. They awakened a powerful wander-lust. She celebrated her twenty-first birthday in Bombay. It was on the power of this event that I had hoped to spend mine there.

Later in the same year, in the winter of 1918, my father and grand-parents were in Shanghai and spent a memorable evening at the home of a wealthy Chinese merchant.

"The silverware at dinner extended for eight inches on either side of the plate. I have never seen so much silver. Your daddy was treated like the most royal guest of all, with little Chinese houseboys in black slip-pers buzzing all around him. They called him 'The Little Master.' The merchant's wife had tiny feet and had to be carried everywhere. Her feet had been bound since she was a young girl. When the evening was over and we were leaving, I noticed the beautiful silk embroidered shoes she wore. They were a lovely shade of magenta, with the most charming flower design embroidered on them. The shoes themselves were so intri-cately sewn with minute stitches, all by hand, of course. The merchant's wife noticed my staring at them, I suppose, and through an interpreter I smiled and told her how pretty her shoes were. Soon after that we gave our thanks and said good-bye.

"Next morning a parcel was delivered to your grandfather on the ship. Do you remember the story? Do you remember what was inside?"

I nodded. Of course I did. When Nana died she left one of the shoes to me and one to Cindy. We reunited them and gave them back to The Little Master.

Nana replaced fear of the unknown with an incentive to take chances. It is not surprising that I grew up with a keenness for adven-tures.

Nana lived in California most of her adult life and never looked back to the country of her birth. She had been brought up on one of the largest farms (which it still is), on the Island of Öland in Sweden, but it was too remote, she said, and difficult to make a comfortable life in such a place. She immigrated to America during the potato famine in the early 1900's, married my grandfather and embraced The Land of Plenty. America was the modern, blessed place, ripe with opportunity for those who applied themselves. Like other immigrants, my grandparents worked hard and were rewarded. America was a different country then, less contrived, with fewer lawyers, less government, and more integrity.

Something very interesting happened when Nana died several years ago. Geoff and I were in New Hampshire with the children that summer. Nana was living in a Christian Science facility in San Francisco, called The Benevolent Association. She was going through a very difficult patch of advanced cervical cancer, but because of her religious convictions, it was not discussed. Her belief was that to discuss it as a physical reality would be to empower the disease. (To me this can be an extremely perilous form of denial. I believe that in terms of healing it is important for most of us to identify the disease and, among other things, to work on the core issues and problems it represents. Then we can claim the blueprint of our divine perfection. Diseases can be clues.)

One night as we lay sleeping, I sat up in bed. "Nana is going to die on a Sunday, and it could be *this* Sunday."

I looked over at the clock. The digital readout was 3:00 a.m. It already was Sunday. Somehow this message wasn't frightening or unsettling at all.

"How like her to choose a Sunday," I remember thinking. She was a very unusual person.

Plumping the bed pillows I struggled to go back to sleep. It wasn't until after sunrise that, on returning to sleep, I vaguely heard one of our houseguests creeping down the creaky wooden stairs.

I awakened at 9:00 or so, having completely forgotten about Nana. It seems peculiar, but the important memory was gone. It had vanished without a trace. We played tennis after breakfast, and at about 11:00 there was a DONG-DONG-DONG on the brass bell at the house. Someone on the court had a telephone call. Geoff ran across the lawn. It was probably a business call.

We were wrong, and he called me in. It was my mother.

"Hi, Mom. How are you?" I could hear a long, sustained breath on the other end. She managed to ask after the children. But Mother rarely called long distance just to say hello.

"What is it?"

"I have some very sad news," she said. "Your Nana passed away last night."

"I know," I heard myself say, and began to cry. "I woke up last night thinking about it. I knew that Nana was going to die on a Sunday and that it could be today."

"You knew?" Mother was surprised. "Daddy was with her from about midnight."

It was as though the news had clicked my antennae onto another channel. After a while I pulled myself together and asked, "When did Nana actually die?"

"She passed away peacefully at about 3:00 a.m."

"I am glad that she won't be in pain anymore."

Then something occurred to me.

"I woke up at 3:00 on our clock; that would be midnight in San Francisco. Strange, isn't it?"

We comforted one another with loving remembrances of the good life that Nana had had. She was the best.

"You know," Mother said, "we spend so much time praying for a good life; then at some point we pray for a good death. Even though Nana had a period of suffering, she died peacefully and fulfilled." Then Mother added, "She loved you very much, you know."

"I do."

Later in the day our houseguest mentioned that he hoped he hadn't awakened any of us as he crept down the stairs so early that morning. "I went off to jog on the beach pretty early," he said. His wife rolled her eyes. "It was about 6:00." The times fit impeccably. It was 3:00 Pacific Standard time.

This comforting retrospective was like a feature movie. It reminded me of how much I loved my grandmother, how special our relationship was, and how she had instilled a sense of adventure in my life.

It would be all right to continue on the voyage now. It wasn't one I would have chosen; it wasn't fun, but it would be all right.

10

Technology...the knack of so arranging the world that we don't have to experience it.

—Max Frisch

As I became physically weaker, it was difficult to feel lucky. Midway through the chemotherapy course I was very tired. My basic features had been modified: I gained weight and sprouted chipmunk cheeks from the steroids, and went from 120 pounds before surgery to 112 pounds after. By February this became 135. The wig made me look like one of Jim Henson's Muppets.

In the grand scheme of things, fatigue had a purpose, though. It became impossible to run around with lists of things to accomplish. The Listaholic took early retirement. I learned how to say "no," and how to allow friends and family to be helpful. My particular role as family linchpin dissolved, never to materialize in quite the same way again, and the need to oversee and orchestrate everything began to fade. I didn't have to be in charge for life to progress smoothly. It wasn't my job to take care of everybody; it had been arrogant and ignorant for me to have thought it was.

Cindy encouraged me to modify my diet. On her well-informed advice and general bullying the amounts of vegetables and fruit were increased, red meat was eliminated entirely, as was nearly all animal fat. The one exception allowed was Peppermint Ice Cream, not then available in fat-free form. It was soothing on the mouth and throat sores, which followed the chemotherapy treatments.

By Christmas I was growing impatient and difficult. Small things became issues.

"Why doesn't this work!" I fumed, ranting over the quality of a mascara. Mother came over and put both of her arms around me and rocked

51

me back and forth as we stood in front of the mirror.

"Sweetie, your eyelashes are nearly all gone," she said, "but they will be back."

It was not an easy period. There were muffled screams in the bath, and frightened sobs when I first saw the intensely bright red veins in my legs, colored by the chemotherapy fluid. It was horrifying.

While all of this was going on, help came in many forms and from many directions. Dear friends, primarily women, passed on information about healing, which they reckoned might be useful. Special groups in Cambridge and Hong Kong routinely put my name in healing circles, a powerful thing to do.

One friend sent a handwritten list of personality traits, which Carl Simonton describes as being commonly held by cancer survivors. Cancer survivors tend to:

- be successful in their careers
- enjoy their careers
- be receptive and creative
- be sometimes hostile/able to be hostile
- have a high degree of self-esteem and self-love
- be rarely docile
- be intelligent and self-reliant
- value interaction with others
- appreciate diversity among friends and acquaintances

There was a hastily written note near the bottom: "Sounds like you!"

But what were the personality traits which had helped to move me into this mess? I had been:

- hypercritical, expecting perfection of myself (and to a lesser extent of others)
- impatient and impatient
- quietly judgmental (like a crusty New Yorker)
- always honoring and responding to the needs of others, while neglecting my own
- living in a world of "shoulds"
- perpetually pressed to accomplish

I had also allowed a handful of relationships to continue in my life, which were harmful and unpleasant. There was a mutual charade of friendliness for the sake of harmony, but these relationships were toxic. Somewhere along the way I had lost a good part of my true self and became a person whose life was dictated excessively by not only the charade, but by the thoughts and needs of others. Ultimately an abundance of negative emotions were hidden deep inside; without knowing it or meaning to, anger and hurt had been stockpiled there.

The good news was that this illness-prone set of patterns and personality had come with an escape ladder. It was around this time that I discovered Joseph Campbell, a masterful guide on the rungs. Campbell had been professor of mythology at Sarah Lawrence College for 38 years. His book, *The Hero with A Thousand Faces*, is a classic work, which explores the spiritual, cultural and mystical development of humankind. The main idea in all of the worlds' mythologies is that there is an invisible plane that supports all we do. My angels and pennies, visions of color, and the unusual miracles I had experienced naturally came to mind.

Another very common theme in mythology is "The Hero's Journey." The hero ventures into the unknown, moving blindly into a mysterious and dangerous abyss. From these life-threatening adventures the hero gleans two crucial elements: experience and knowledge. She/he survives the event and returns to the community with new energy and vision. This was a fine concept. I embraced it and decided to be a hero. It was better than remaining an ignorant fool.

Campbell also relates a tale from the Arthurian Legends in which The Holy Grail appears to the Knights of The Round Table. Sir Gawain rises with a toast and calls the knights into action:

"Let us go forth in search of The Holy Grail," he proclaims.

The Knights agree, but with one significant caveat. Each must enter a dark place in the forest and follow an untrodden path. In other words, every knight must take the most difficult way, and he must travel alone.

In applying this story to my own situation, I found comfort. There was a sporadic, sometimes capricious quality to my journey. I frequently criticized myself for being a typical Gemini, jumping from one idea to the next, reading five books at a time, trying to grasp and synthesize them all. But crucial in this process was learning to surrender, to accept help from others, to give up control, and most importantly, to trust where I was being led. Healers, books, seminars, crystals and friends helped illuminate the dark place in the forest. There was tremendous support from the invisible world.

Joseph Campbell helped me to see myself as a prospective hero, a good upwardly mobile move. Sitting at The Round Table, with a silver goblet of wine or a Kir Royale, I was the only female knight, with a wig, and without eyelashes, but as brave as the best of them. They accepted me. It was a very good image to hold.

At about this time I also discovered a fine healer in Pleasant Hill, California. Connie Kinney discovered her gift while working at a counseling center. On one occasion Connie was asked if she would just put her hands on an ailing female client's back; when she did this, all of the back pain left.

"At first," Connie explained, "I thought whatever healing took place was just a coincidence. I was also a bit frightened. However, I continued to practice on all of those who worked in the center."

Twelve years later, Connie became a consultant and began practicing healing full time. I have since come to know outstanding healers from all over the world, but Connie was a lovely and phenomenal first exposure.

It is her belief that through her practices she simply encourages the life force in others, helping it to be awakened, expanded, and perhaps most significantly, unblocked. Connie never studied Reiki, but she uses her hands in much the same way as a Reiki practitioner. Soothing heat emanates from her palms, and what can only be described as the presence of great love fills her treatment room.

In the beginning the greatest obvious benefit was in learning how to release stress and fear. I would lie down on a padded table with a blanket and, with Connie's guidance, become quiet inside. She would then sense my energy, moving her hands in a wave-like motion. This is a movement which many healers employ.

"What does it feel like?" I asked.

"Like gentle water currents," she answered.

Then she might say, "Your energy is great today," or "try to get a little more rest. You feel tired."

Connie taught me how to monitor ordinary feelings more carefully and make them an integral part of my being. After a few visits I told her about the mysterious pennies and asked what she thought. Her eyes twinkled and she smiled.

"How do you *feel* when you find them?" she asked.

"I feel loved. I feel less alone. But it has been going on for so long, it is crazy making. I am curious and frustrated. Where do they come from?"

"The pennies are wonderful. That's all you really need to know for now. Just accept them with gratitude."

I later sought her advice on applying to Stanford for a bone marrow evaluation. She had an opinion, but wouldn't give it. Through prayer and meditation I would have to discover the answer for myself. Prayer is asking; meditation is listening. If I asked, the answer was supposed to come. It did. I decided not to go to Stanford.

When Connie worked with me, memories of childhood came without prompting. Sometimes I cried, afterward feeling bathed in light and love. Tears release stress hormones and provide a great cleansing for our bodies as well as our souls. It is health enhancing to cry.

Connie helped me to discern which relationships called for greater compassion and which required "tough love." She very gently dispelled the vigorous code of blind obedience toward elders, which I was brought up to serve whether I respected them, or not.

Selflessness was yet another misguided personal value. I saw a hand printed tee shirt in Manila two years ago, which describes this well:

> If you think the world is sick
> Begin with your own life and heal it.
> Once we heal our own lives
> The world won't be sick anymore.

If we spend all of our time on others, we miss the point of our own lives. It has been said that we become human *doings* rather than human *beings*. Selflessness can also be a form of procrastination. We may choose never to take time for ourselves, because the self is the most difficult and scary part to look at. If we don't pay attention and respond to ourselves, our personal lessons will be repeated again and again. Simultaneously the Universe will keep turning up the volume and raising the stakes until we respond. The old personality and life style won't leave us with a lot of options. To become well again we have to go through the dark place in the forest and learn to heal our lives. At first, when willing, all we want is a full set of directions.

"Give me a map. I want to get out of here!"

"At least give me instructions so I can find the way!"

Guess what: There aren't any instructions, and there isn't any map. That is the challenge. By divine design we are meant to fly blind. In the absence of a plan we are forced to relinquish control, to cease living in old ways, old ruts. Eventually, in the most healthful of scenarios, there is surrender, giving in on the part of our powerfully controlling egos. Once we are able to acknowledge that Someone or Something far greater is in charge, we gain humility. It is in that instant that we connect with a far greater, inordinately more helpful power. With this shift of consciousness, there is so much of life that becomes positive. It becomes possible to trust the Process and the Operator, even when the situation looks bleak. It is possible to recognize the stranger on the street as a fellow traveler with his/her own unique itinerary.

11

*Human beings are first and foremost energy beings.
Everyone has an energy counterpart which both occupies
the body and extends beyond it as the aura. It is this
which supplies life, health and vitality to the physical
body. When the energy system breaks down or is blocked
in any way, related parts of the body cease to vibrate with
life force and this creates ill-health...*

—Betty Shine, *Mind to Mind*

The chemotherapy treatments were over in March, and I returned to Hong Kong.

Hong Kong is tough, spirited, and fast moving, a city of hyperactivity and neon real estate in the sky. The brilliant hot lights give the city a pulse of frenetic excitement. The Chinese often compare Hong Kong with San Francisco as two enchanting, irresistible women. Hong Kong, the older of the two, is accomplished and sophisticated, wealthy and romantically sexy. San Francisco is lovely too, but more like an adolescent ready to bloom.

On our return I wondered if it would be possible to step back from the pulsating life of the city and find a quiet niche. I was so easily tired that guided tours for distant relatives or friends were no longer possible; fairly routine dinner parties for 24 were impossible to think of. I hoped we wouldn't be so removed from the old life as to feel like outsiders. Fortunately friends were magnanimously supportive and these demands fell quietly away.

On following Lawrence Stoller's advice, I wrote to Lazaris, asking for a telephone consultation. An appointment was made for May 6th. We waited with great anticipation. I wanted to know Lazaris' opinion about the bone marrow transplant. Having decided against it, had this been the best decision?

The following is an excerpt from our conversation on May 6, 1990.

Lynne: Last September I had two lymphoma tumors removed from my abdominal area. I completed six months of chemotherapy. I was then encouraged to go to Stanford [Medical School] to talk to a team of doctors who are very involved in bone marrow transplants. I felt I wouldn't need such a treatment, but wondered if it might be smart for me to have some "insurance." My husband and my father-in-law were also encouraging me to go and see the Stanford group. So I thought, should I have some bone marrow taken out and stored? I did a lot of prayerful asking within myself, and ultimately felt it might not be a wise approach for me to take.

Am I wise to avoid the bone marrow transplant? Or should I cover all the bases? Should I be more experienced in visualization or with methods like Reiki before following this less-conventional approach?

I would also like to know where I am on my journey and what I can do to enhance the joy I find along the way.

Lazaris: All right, Lynne, certainly so. We will look at a number of issues here.

First, your decision not to have the bone marrow extracted was the correct one. That kind of "insurance" was unnecessary. This sort of thing is only to be done in very dire situations. We congratulate you for being able to understand this, for doing the right thing.

Each person creates their own reality, and it is important to understand that you had the opportunity to use allopathic medicines to your advantage. We would suggest that you were right to use them; this is something that cannot be ignored.

We are often asked the question, "Where does one's responsibility begin and end?" In Eastern thought, if a child falls out of a boat into a river, that's karma. [But there's] the question: Should you jump in and save them? Or should you let them go ahead and drown?

We would suggest, jump in and save them. The child fell into the river all right, but they fell into the river in front of *you*. If they really wanted to die, they could figure out a way to do so when you weren't around.

And so, you have created two lymphomas in the abdominal region; but you have done it at a time in history when beneficial medications are available.

The most advisable thing for you at the time was to have the lymphoma removed, followed up by chemotherapy. You went through this with relative ease, with minimal side effects. This speaks very positively to your intent to survive and be healthy.

You could also have had a bone marrow transplant, but you said, "No, that's where I draw the line." So now we would use alternative healing approaches.

OK, what's this lymphoma cancer about? The lymphatic system dumps the garbage of the body. When you develop a lymphoma what you are telling yourself is, "I am carrying too many emotional toxins, more than my lymph glands can handle, more than the system can process. And therefore the garbage is backing up."

An organized metropolitan area like Hong Kong has a way to process garbage. If everybody all of a sudden had too much garbage and the garbage trucks couldn't pick it up in one day, it would start backing up. This is just what happens with the body. The sewage treatment plant inside your body got overloaded. It backed up and therefore created all these health problems.

So what do you need to do? You say, "I'm not going to be a martyr here. I will also work with what these toxins are."

In your case, Lynne, there are tremendous amounts of hurt. You have learned to process the anger, but the hurt is still foreign to you. It is very frightening to really get in touch with that. It is scary because you say to yourself, "Good grief! I can't stand self-pitying people. People who whine just drive me crazy. I wouldn't want to look like that. So I won't let myself express the hurt."

Also Lynne, you are afraid to lose control. There is a part of you that says, "Look, I can deal with anger. But hurt? I might get stuck there. I might not be able to get out, and that would be a fine kettle of fish."

In processing tremendous amounts of anger your health has improved substantially. The hurt is old stuff from the earliest of childhood; and we would suggest that there is also hurt from other lifetimes. The key at this point is to start releasing some of this. Go back to when you were five to eight, also when you were 14 to 16.

The way you do it is basically to set up a time. Say to yourself, "This evening between 8:00 and 8:30 I am going to release the hurt. I'll start talking about it; I'll start running it through my mind; I'll start letting myself feel the pain of it, roll around on the floor, if that's what it takes. I let myself curl up in a little ball on the bed and sob. I let myself feel sorry for myself, if need be, to prime the pump. Once 8:30 is here, time's up! I'm going to do something that I really enjoy, take a lovely bath perhaps. Reward myself when the time is up and I need to shift the mood." Do this exercise periodically.

I would also talk to the little girl and ask her to tell me about the hurt she feels. As you become empathetic with her, the hurt will be released.

This in conjunction with the work you have already been doing can put you over the edge. Then you will know you have this thing beat.

It's not a matter of greater visualization; it's just a matter of greater focus. If you could get over your particular resistances, you could clear this cancer quite effectively.

We would suggest in the larger scope that you continue to work with visualization and with Reiki. For keeping health in the body and preventing illness, we like Reiki a lot. It is self-done and you don't have to rely on others.

You also ask: "Where am I going?" We would suggest that first of all you are in a very good place. This cancer has been a very beneficial catalyst. You have really "cleaned up your act" as you call it in your vernacular. You have cleared out a tremendous amount of the stuff of the past, and that's superb. You have done brilliant work.

Also you are becoming more and more an inspiration to others. This is part of what you want to do in this lifetime. Thus, we would suggest that you are coming into your own.

There are five additional [things] you have to hold your focus on.

One is leadership. You came in as a woman, and women are not afforded that position automatically. You have to earn it, even *overearn* it. We would suggest that you are here to inspire, to uplift, to teach, and in your own way to heal. And that is what you do: you give a tremendous amount of energy, a tremendous amount of hope. "By golly! I can do it. I have spent the afternoon with this woman, Lynne Picard, and I don't know what happened, but..." In that sense you are a leader.

The second focus is communication, and this is one of your strengths: the ability to communicate something new. You express your creativity as a jack-of-all-trades. You paint a little, you write a little, you do some design work, and you do any number of things superbly, because you have a tremendous range. You don't like small talk; you find it rather tedious, rather boring and rather irritating. This is because you are interested in real communication.

The third focus is service to humanity. Your life is a journey. You help people change the way they think, and you will be of service in this larger scope.

The problem with service, Lynne, is that it is a narrow roadway and people can fall off to two sides. You have seen those who fall into martyrhood, and end up being used by those they are trying to serve. These people end up ruining their lives because of their blind dedication. People who get involved in human rights, for example, can often hurt their families.

The other problem is arrogance: those who feel superior to people they are serving. In that sense they do more damage than good. The point is that you are here to find the balance between the two.

Finally you are here to work with love, to learn through love, the ups and downs, the ins and outs, the backs and forths. You want to know what might be called "the many faces of love," how love develops with friends, acquaintances, business people, and to experience its many aspects.

You wonder why you can't settle down, why you always want more out of your relationships, but as you understand the focus of these relationships, it is going to work out very nicely.

The last focus is power. You are here to learn about power. Again, as a woman you're going to have to build. Males are given power automatically, whether they want it or not. Yet we would say that you are now moving into your own. Within another year you are going to feel a certain sense of accomplishment, of "I've done it! I feel the leadership, the communication, the service, the love and the power." Then there will be a whole new surge of energy, almost like booster rockets throwing you into a whole new orbit. Your fifth decade is going to be really a very exciting time, devoted to a lot of very highly creative projects; a lot of them are going to be very inspiring of creativity in others.

You are on the brink of some very important changes that look very powerful and very positive.

We close with love and peace.

12

You! You whom we love...
You do not see us.
You do not hear us.
You imagine us in the far distance...
Yet we are so near.
We are the messengers who bring closeness to those in
the distance.
We are not the message...
We are the messengers.
The message is love.
We are nothing.
You are everything to us.
Let us dwell in your eyes!
See your world through us.
Recapture through us that loving look once again.
Then we'll be close to you...
And you to him.

> —Spoken by the Angels Raphaela and Cassiel
> in the German film, *Far Away, So Close*,
> Grand Jury prizewinner, Cannes, 1993

In the summer of 1990 we returned to Lake Tahoe. I took joy and found relief in the high country, easing into a quiet routine in which I could grow strong again. The mysterious pennies still appeared. The most memorable of them turned up in August.

We had packed a lunch of sandwiches and cookies and apples, having decided to take an easy hike up to one of the small alpine lakes.

It was a majestic day, an ideal mix of hot sun, cool pine-shaped shadows and robin's egg blue skies. The trail was dusty and the air was dry. Everyone looked forward to the locally famous fresh lemonade sold from a small cabin at our destination. Geoff and Peter discussed whether or not they would dive off the 50' rock. In spite of a longstanding drought, Lake Angora was still plenty deep, but the length of the dive had been extended.

Our little party arrived at the lake, feeling both at home and freshly in awe, as though we were seeing it for the first time. It was always like this. Geoff rummaged through his rucksack in search of change to buy lemonade, while I set about arranging a striped beach towel, which would be our picnic table on the sand.

Flinging the towel out, it moved on a gentle breeze and landed flat, with just one corner curled up. Bending down to make it straight, I caught a glimpse of what looked like a tiny piece of copper wire. It was exactly at the specific point of the maverick corner. Without thinking, I reached for it.

It was a penny that had been buried in the sand, standing on its thin edge. I picked it up and started to cry. By now there was no wondering about coincidences. Who were these angels at work? What was going on? Whatever they were, they were pretty sensational. Standing at an altitude of 7,500 feet in the middle of a pristine wilderness, whatever was going on had my respect. I could sense tenacity as well as humor. It was the most creatively placed penny of all, unforgettable. My tears responded to the message, "We are still here. We love you, and we aren't relaxing yet." For a brief moment there was a cool draft on the back of my neck, and I remember wondering about it.

When August ended, we routinely returned to Hong Kong; Lex and Peter went back to Massachusetts.

In September we were invited to the birthday party of a friend who is married to one of Geoff's Harvard classmates. It was a wonderful evening, with dinner on an outside terrace, looking onto Hong Kong's magnificent harbor. For me, the most important conversation didn't come until the end. As we were leaving, this lovely lady, the birthday child, took me to one side.

"After what you went through last year," she said, "I want to give you something." She struggled and searched for casual, reassuring words. "You probably won't need this, but just in case, I want to give you the name of my mother's healer in the Philippines."

"What has happened to your mother?"

"It is an old story by now. She had very bad sinus headaches for over 12 years. She went to a lot of specialists all over America and in Canada, but nobody could help her. The headaches kept coming. Finally a friend in Manila introduced her to Gary Magno. He healed her, and she hasn't had one of her headaches since."

"Who is Gary Magno?" I asked.

"A psychic healer."

"Is he one of those people who reaches inside of you and takes things out of your body?"

"Yes. No anesthesia, no pain, no scars." Her voice was more hushed.

"Does it really work? It's hard to believe." My eyes were wide open, forehead wrinkled with curiosity.

"If you go to one of the real healers, and there are several of them, it does work. The problem is that most of the people who claim to be psychic healers are frauds. They use chicken parts and animal blood. You really have to be careful. These people put the good healers in question, and there is a lot of suspicion about it. But Gary has helped a lot of people. My Mother and her friends feel that he is incredible."

The note with Gary's information on it was put into a catchall drawer in an old Chinese armoire for safekeeping. Just in case.

A week later a prescription came in the mail for estrogens, which had been recommended by the team of doctors who had been so helpful in California. After the chemotherapy treatments my estrogen level was very low, and the doctors felt that a hormone replacement regimen would be a good idea. Within the next few days I took the prescription to The Victoria Dispensary, a wonderful old-fashioned drugstore in Central, and handed it to one of the pharmacists.

"Hello," I smiled at the man, "could you fill this for me, please?" The young Chinese man studied the piece of paper for a very long time. Something was wrong. They were probably out of stock. It happens in Hong Kong, or else they didn't carry this particular American medicine and would have to substitute.

"This is a prescription from a doctor outside of Hong Kong?" he asked.

"Yes. It is from an internist in California."

"I am very sorry," he said, "but we can't fill this. You must have this prescription rewritten by a Hong Kong registered doctor." After a moment he added, "It's the law, you see."

"Oh no," I said quietly. Another doctor was the last thing I wanted.
The pharmacist felt bad.

"You can imagine," he said, "anybody could come to Hong Kong and have a prescription pad printed. We would have no way of knowing who was a doctor and who wasn't. So we just deal with doctors who are registered. I can't do you a favor, in this case."

It made sense.

"Just take it to any hospital Emergency Room. Do you have a hospital near where you live?"

"Yes, The Matilda," I answered.

"The doctor on duty will sign it over for you. They do it all the time."

"I will. Thank you for your help." I waved and was off.

A few days later I went along to The Matilda Hospital, and explained the situation to a clerk.

"Please take a seat," she said, in halting English. "Dr. A. will be with you in a few minutes."

Soon after that I was sitting in the doctor's office explaining my situation.

"Of course I will sign the prescription over," she said. "I am going to reduce the dosage, though, because I feel it is twice as much as you need."

As she wrote, I thanked her and began gathering up my things.

"Could I just examine your abdomen before you leave?"

I took a deep breath, and with all of my clothes on, climbed onto the examining table.

She loosened my skirt and began to probe the abdominal area, returning to one place again and again. She had a growing look of concern on her face, which was frightening.

"I don't want to alarm you," she said, "but I think you should have another scan. Right away."

"Today?" I asked in disbelief.

"I will order one for you."

"What do you feel?"

"A lump," she said. "It feels like a golf ball that's been run over by a truck. It might be nothing. Let's do the scan and find out for sure."

"Oh no." It was back to the place of silent screams.

I went upstairs to the C-T Scan Unit, handed the doctor's order to the Chinese nurse on duty and asked if I could use the telephone. I wanted to call Geoff.

There were eight people or more sitting in the waiting room when the nurse brusquely banged the old-fashioned 1940s black telephone atop the counter and went on with her work. I took more deep breaths and dialed Geoff at the office.

"Hi Sweetie." Then there was a long composure-gathering pause. "I'm in an awful mess." From then on it was a slow, choking conversation, tears ebbing and flowing through horrible memories and sensations, trying not to cry.

"Where are you?" Geoff asked.

"At The Matilda," I said. I explained why and what had happened. "The doctor on duty wants me to have a C-T Scan right away."

The nurse overheard our conversation and inserted herself loudly into it.

"No scan until we have a check from you," she said. And then, pointing to the receiver, "Tell him. Tell him."

I wanted to leave.

"You can't just walk in and have a scan," Geoff reminded me. You need to drink the tracing material well in advance. Remember?"

"Yes. Of course I do." Finally I said, "I am walking out of here now. This doesn't feel right."

"Good," Geoff said. "Let's find out where else you can go."

"I know where I am going already, and I really hope you'll come with me."

"Where?" Geoff asked.

"To Manila."

He didn't miss a beat. "How can I help?"

"Could you have someone call Gary Magno's office in Manila and get an appointment? Someone who can speak Tagalog in case they don't speak English?"

Geoff hesitated. Then he said, "Sure. I can try. I don't think we will be able to get an appointment by this weekend, though."

The plan felt right. "Let's see," I said. "If it is the thing to do, I think it will fall into place. Will you try?"

"Of course," he said. "I'll get on it right now."

With enormous pleasure I asked the officious nurse to cancel the order and walked out. Within the hour Geoff called me at home.

"We have an appointment on Saturday and Sunday, too, if it is necessary. We'll get the Saturday morning Cathay flight. The tickets are in the works. One more thing: I love you."

13

Miracles do not happen in contradiction to nature, but only in contradiction of that which is known to us in nature.

—St. Augustine

On October 6, we walked to the Cathay Pacific gate for the Manila flight, the gate most distant from the Immigration Section. There were two middle aged women and a man ahead of us; they were going to Manila, too. As we neared the boarding area, a shiny brass button hit the black rubberized floor. It must have come off one of their sweaters, or perhaps off the gentleman's blazer. I put my luggage down and stooped to retrieve it for them, but they walked on without taking any notice. In fact, it wasn't a brass button at all. It was a very bright new Hong Kong fifty-cent piece.

We arrived Saturday morning and found the city baked in a dirty industrial heat haze. There was more poverty and squalor, more disorganization than there had been under the corrupt Marcos regime. The city had drastically deteriorated. As the country worked at redefining itself under new leadership, there seemed to be a weakened spirit and a loss of national identity and pride.

The long, gracious palm-lined boulevard that follows The Bay of Manila was now strewn with rubbish and the island full of splotchy grass. It appeared as though some flea-bitten animal had moved in where country club lawns used to grow. Small children were begging in the traffic jams, often in pairs, a little one on the cocked hip of an elder sister, with outstretched hands and glassy eyes. I had seen these eyes in India years before. In hopelessness the spirit and vigor of these small bodies had gone somewhere else. There was a vacancy. Teenage boys with brown teeth sold chewing gum and cigarettes from wooden boxes strapped around their necks; others hawked flower garlands and newspapers.

This seemed a peculiar place for miracles, a forgotten place.

I began second-guessing in earnest, dancing between instinct and logic. Was I acting out of desperation or following my angels? Was it providential that a very good friend had given Gary Magno's name and address to me? And just ten days before I needed it? Wasn't there at least some indication of divine direction? I wasn't sure. And what about the appointment on such short notice? Whatever the truth was, it seemed a far better plan to try Gary Magno's healing sessions than to return to America for another round of chemotherapy.

We arrived at the hotel before the appointment. We dropped our bags, registered, and got a taxi to The Healing Center, which was located in a residential section of Manila, very near the sea. In its day, this had been a pleasant residential area, but now it was a slum.

There was an entrance off the street, with teak parquet floors, very basic furniture, a receptionist's desk, and an enormous television, much larger than anything we had at home. Upstairs was a good-sized waiting room with rows of chrome-frame chairs with shiny vinyl seats. Electric fans were mounted strategically on the walls along with religious statuary and paintings of Christian saints. Playing on the tape deck as we entered was a Siddha Yoga Chant, which I had heard in Hong Kong, "Om Namah Shivayah." After that came a Hallelujah hymn. One would have thought that this would have been more of a Catholic place.

Gary is a quietly shy and graceful man of Spanish ancestry. When he arrived, all of us who had come for healing joined hands and sang hymns and chants. The level of sincerity and humility mixed with desperation was evident. Most of us had lines of tears running down our faces; we were without masks or protective egos, all hoping for miracles. There was a powerful atmosphere in the waiting room, a sense of what I can only describe as a divine connection. None of us felt separate from the other. Gary then said a prayer and we joined him later in The Lord's Prayer. After that everyone sat down and waited.

Terry, Gary's wife, sat down beside me. She was a striking strawberry blonde, shy but forthright and supportive of her husband's healing. She was an American from Anchorage. We hadn't needed to speak Tagalog at all.

"Why are you here?" she asked.

"Because I have a problem in my abdominal area," I replied (not mentioning specifically the findings of the doctor at the Matilda Hospital).

"Well, you look wonderful!" she said. "We can usually tell by looking at the eyes, and yours are radiant."

"I am moving in that direction," I said, "but I don't think I'm there yet. I had cancer and chemotherapy last year."

"I can't believe it," she said incredulously. "You really do look well. Do you know why you got sick in the first place?"

"Yes," I said, "I think I do." It was evident that this was not a medical question.

"And have you dealt with it?" she went on. "You need to or you will get sick again."

"You are right."

"So have you?" she reiterated.

"Mostly. I think I have about 10%-15% more to do." (A naïve measurement, this assessment was miles off the mark.)

"Well, keep at it," she said, "don't think you can coast or procrastinate."

There was some activity behind a large glass window that separated the healing room from the waiting room. The blue draperies, which hung on the window, were now opened, presenting a sort of theatre behind glass. There was an elevated table inside, lots of pictures of Jesus, a signed photograph of The Pope, mixed with Chamber of Commerce Awards, and fluorescent lighting. It was surreal.

"Should my husband come with me?" I asked.

Terry turned to Geoff, and with a very serious expression asked, "Do you think this faith healing is possible? Do you have an open mind about it?"

"Yes." Geoff's response was immediate, a surprise which made me glad.

"Then it will be all right for you to come in," she said. "Lynne will be glad for your support." She gave me a reassuring hug, and then moved on to speak to someone else.

A Chinese-Filipino gentleman, who had spent his professional life as a medical doctor, came into the waiting room, accompanied by three generations of family. He was in his early 80's and shuffled with frailty, arms stiffly immobile, like an old soldier stooping slightly, but permanently at attention.

His hair, or what was left of it, gave him the look of a cancer patient. His demeanor was angry and helpless. He had a brain tumor, classified as inoperable. His most prized granddaughter, also a doctor, was in Boston, teaching at a medical school there. Her specialty was neurology.

This granddaughter had put together a global medical council that meticulously reviewed his case. Their judgment was, "We cannot help you. You need a miracle." His granddaughter suggested, "Why don't you find the best faith healer in Manila and go to him for help? You have nothing to lose."

It was easy to see that the poor man felt God had punished him unjustly. Visiting a faith healer pierced his dignity and was an affront to his training, to everything he knew. It was insulting, causing him to lose respect for himself as a medical practitioner. We could hear him telling Terry in a very emotional state that he had led a decent life, loving his family, close to God, and being of service to others. Terry held him and calmed him down. She was wonderful. By the time the older gentleman was led into the healing room his anger seemed to have lessened, and he was far more at ease.

A pair of young Swedish journalists positioned themselves with their cameras, ready to record the healing. For me this added a carnival-like atmosphere which, though I watched it, was upsetting. They had come because a well-known Swedish actor, diagnosed with terminal cancer, had been cured after seeing Gary, and was now leading a very normal life. It was in all the newspapers in Stockholm. The journalists had come to do a follow-up story.

We watched with uncomfortable fascination as Gary first "x-rayed" the elderly doctor by holding a clean white sheet in front of him. When he looked through it, diseased or dead tissue would appear as dark shapes, although none of this was visible to us.

One of Gary's assistants gave the man a cross to hold and told him to pray. As he lay there, Gary worked quickly making "incisions" with his fingers. Impossible as it sounds his fingers actually entered the man's body. Blood squirted as he pulled out diseased or unhealthy tissue. His assistants wiped him off with clean towels.

The old man moaned loudly, and seemed physically and emotionally jarred by each new entry of Gary's fingers. I wondered if he was in pain, or if he was simply terrified. The shutters on the Swedes' cameras clicked away with great speed.

After five minutes or so, Gary went to work on the brain tumor. Incredible as it sounds, he actually took a small piece of it out through the skull. (I later learned that if the entire tumor had been removed at once, the man would have died. Gary took it out in stages over a period of weeks.)

This first procedure lasted only 15 minutes. The elderly doctor was helped off the table, his family dressed and lovingly held him. Then he was ushered away.

A pair of older twins, ladies from Seattle with gray permed hair, came next.

"We come once a year," one of them told me.

"It is our vacation," said the other. "Gary 'cleans us up and clears us out.'"

"It is a new and better kind of health insurance," they added together in Tweedle Dum and Tweedle Dee style. Then they laughed.

The two of them went in together and undressed by turn. The first sister was cleaned and cleared in what seemed a pretty fast, routine exercise, taking bits of tissue from around her throat and near her heart. The second lady had her left eye operated on and was quite swollen afterward. We never knew what Gary had done. It didn't seem appropriate to ask. Both ladies were extremely pleased and said they would be back the next day.

A Filipina went next, a woman with a very large growth protruding from her neck. I supposed it was a goiter, but perhaps it was a tumor. Gary went through the same process, releasing a yellow oozing substance. After that I couldn't watch anymore.

When my turn came, I asked if the journalists could leave and the draperies be closed. As a modest person, the open arena made me uncomfortable. Gary arranged it and Geoff helped me to undress. I stood behind the white "x-ray" sheet and was also given a cross to hold.

Gary said a quiet prayer to himself, and looked through the sheet for the "black places." I climbed onto the table with just my panties on and was asked to lie down, to relax and to pray.

Without knowing about the doctor's examination in Hong Kong, Gary went immediately to the spot she had found, and took out a tumor. Blood splattered half way across the room; I could feel the warmth of it squirting out of my body and onto my legs and arms as the attendants wiped me down with damp cloths. Gary nudged me to open my eyes. Then he held the tumor up for me to see. It was shaped like a squashed golf ball, perhaps a bit smaller in size.

Next he went into the base of my throat and cleaned out more material. He ran one short fingernail lightly along the length of both legs, releasing what looked like clotting blood. As he moved to work on my left ovary, I panicked. There was another incision.

"Only a cyst," he said. "You will be more comfortable without it." (I did have a cyst there, but had forgotten about it. It was painless most of the time.)

He then said another prayer and helped me up, off of the table. As I wrapped the sheet around me, he said, "God bless you."

Full of tears I hugged him. "God bless you, too."

This was a phenomenal experience. Ushered back into the small dressing room, I was to put my clothes on. There wasn't a scar or mark on any part of me. Geoff and I were in shock. We just looked at each other, asking questions with our eyes. Soon locked together in an embrace, both in tears, it was an incredibly moving experience.

In a few minutes an attendant came and nicely asked if I could free the room for the next patient. We were taking too long. I dressed quickly and went back to the waiting room. The operation had taken 20 minutes. I was given a small flask of bottled spring water to drink.

"Sit quietly and rest," Terry said in soft tones. "Your result was very good. You are so receptive," she said. "In an hour or two Gary will take you for another treatment. That will be enough for today."

There was a lot I wanted to say, but all I could manage was, "Thank you," and a long hug.

After a little more than an hour, I went back onto the table. Gary cleaned out more material, small pieces of tissue. He went into a spot near my aorta and removed what looked like clotting blood. I wondered if it was related to the cholesterol problem that I had had since the chemotherapy treatments.

When it was over we went back into the waiting room to rest a little before getting a taxi back to The Manila Hotel. It was just after 4:00 in the afternoon.

Terry came with another bottle of spring water.

"Remember," she said, "you have just had the equivalent of several operations. You must take it easy, and drink plenty of water. Move slowly and don't pick up anything heavy, including the suitcases when you leave tomorrow." Geoff and I looked at each other, nodding in agreement.

"More than anything I would like to take a bath," I said.

"That will be fine," she said, "but don't make it too hot, and don't fall asleep in it," Terry continued. "I want to give you some herbs, too. If there is any chance of infection, they will prevent it. Can you come in again tomorrow morning?"

"Yes, we can," Geoff said. "Our flight back to Hong Kong doesn't leave until the afternoon."

"Good. I will give you some Seven Mountains Tea in the morning. It is a Philippine cleansing remedy which will wash away cells that have been disturbed, the ones that you don't want."

As soon as we got back to the hotel, I drew a deep bath. Neither of us could put the scene out of our minds; we kept repeating the same string of superlative adjectives and adverbs.

A few hours later, not wanting to wander far, we went to The Cowrie

Restaurant in the Manila Hotel for dinner. It was there that we really began to talk about the day.

"What did it feel like?" Geoff asked.

"I could feel pressure, but it didn't hurt. It was only uncomfortable when Gary worked on my throat."

"There were scattered drops of blood squirting everywhere," Geoff said. "I got some on my polo shirt."

"I could feel it squirting. It was warm and smelled like menstrual blood. Maybe that's why I couldn't get a bath soon enough."

"Can you believe after what you went through that we are sitting here having a great dinner? And you can eat anything you want? Let's order a special bottle of wine." Geoff flagged down a waiter.

"I know!" I said, "No tubes, no stitches, not even a mark." It was beyond remarkable.

We moved through three courses, trying to keep our voices down. Ultimately it was impossible to speak of anything else. Each time one of us would try to change the subject we would be powerfully drawn back to the healing room.

"How does he do it?"

"What do you think?"

"Does he have a special relationship with God?"

We took turns scratching our heads, asking the same question in dozens of ways, attempting to move the whole experience into some realm of believability.

"He must have some kind of chemicals in his fingers;" or, "he just has a special gift."

"How do you feel about the miracles in *The Bible* now?" I asked.

"Less allegorically," was Geoff's answer.

"You know," I added, "Beth Gray, a Reiki Grand Master, told me that Reiki healing energy was probably used by Jesus. It seems very plausible now. Gary said that Jesus guides his healing hands, and that he is present in the healing room."

By the time dessert came, the first prize explanation was evident: Gary must be an alien.

"Is it possible that he is from another planet?" Geoff mused.

"Maybe from another galaxy."

"Yes," we agreed, nodding simultaneously. "That is probably it."

There it was, a nice little comfortable cubbyhole in which to file the experiences which were beyond our understanding.

As we undressed for bed, I sensed that there had been a definite shift in consciousness both for myself and for Geoff. My perspective on ordinary life had been dramatically jarred. Things which had seemed so important were trivial now. My personal healing process was phenomenal. When we turned out the lights I said good night to this day with abundant, overflowing thanks, and closed my eyes, looking forward to a deep, regenerative sleep.

A color appeared once again on my mental screen, this time a vibrant rose pink rectangle. I watched it for a few moments to see if there was anything more to come: Any Peter Max fried blue eggs or pussywillows? Walt Disney paint? But there was nothing more. Blinking hard to see if the color would disappear, I found that it didn't. Trying to shake it off, I opened my eyes completely. Then something frightening happened. The rose pink rectangle moved and was "sitting" on the chair over by the window. It appeared to be almost lounging there, bent at the middle, all four corners rounded. I blinked again. This was beyond belief.

It isn't real, I thought. It must be the effect of the image that remains after looking at a light bulb. I blinked harder to see if it would go away. It didn't move at all.

By now Geoff was snoring his sleeping song. I wanted so much to awaken him.

Look, Sweetie! Can you see the bright pink light sitting on the chair? But I couldn't bring myself to do it. He had been through enough stretching experiences for one day. We both had.

So I watched the pink light alone, with the bedclothes tucked up under my chin, perfectly still.

After a few minutes or so, the color simply vanished. It didn't get up and walk away, or sail into the night through a window, it disappeared. Suddenly braver, I sat up in bed and laughed at having been afraid. But what if the brightly colored form had somehow wanted to speak or to touch me? What if it had become ghostly and put on a face?

We returned to the Healing Clinic the following morning. From the back of the waiting room there was a very bold, husky noise. It sounded like, "Oy!" and again, "Oy!"

Everyone turned around to see the elderly Filipino doctor. He wanted to show us something, his arms, which had been immobile yesterday. Once he gained our attention he miraculously flopped them up and down, up and down; then he smiled happily and shuffled in. Everything seemed pretty routine after that.

14

The highest point a man can attain is not knowledge, or virtue, or victory, but something even greater, more heroic and more despairing: sacred awe!

—Nikos Kazantzakis

When Geoff and I returned to Hong Kong we were once again different people. The experience in Manila had moved both of us to another world. The filter through which I, especially, had seen and experienced daily life, was altogether changed. It happens that way. Without fanfare or judgment, it was obvious that the great noise of my everyday life was unnecessary busyness, chasing superficial achievements like a mad listoholic. Had I been the CEO of General Motors it would have been, in principle, the same. The experience with Gary Magno was life altering.

When we lived in Japan I remember in moments of frustration thinking of its culture in a deprecatory way as "The Ant Farm." Standing at the top of one of the wide allees, O-Mote-Sando, one could see the action, as waves of dark-haired people moved along briskly and purposefully, driven by a combination of cultural momentum and accomplishment. Office hours were infamously long in Tokyo; time spent with wives and children was negligible. After the visit to Manila this image and memory came back like a flash with the harsh realization that I was an ant as well, caught up in accomplishment and busyness. My own emotional and spiritual growth had been perpetually held in check for an apparent lack of time.

As the medium in Massachusetts had explained years before, I was giving myself away to too many jobs in too many directions. Modern sages call this "substitute giving." One neglects the giving of time and thought to oneself, but feels (artificially) fulfilled by giving to others. In the Western world Americans are especially proficient at this. For me this substitute giving had become not only a habit, but possibly a place to hide. On any given day I would write down twice as many jobs as I could ever hope to accomplish, pressing myself without mercy, playing the game of "doing more, doing more," and piling on more after that. Life was one constant activity, and I was a slightly frenetic drone moving toward exhaustion. Once I saw this truth for myself, it was all around me.

As Lama Govinda, a German teacher of Tibetan Buddhism, put it when he was alive, "...We have not yet achieved mastery over ourselves, our inner life, our psychic and spiritual forces, in short the dormant faculties of our deeper consciousness. [These forces,] after all, created the world in which we live and all that we have achieved in the form of manifold civilizations. These faculties permit us to see the fundamental oneness of life, the interrelatedness of all peoples and civilizations, and the ultimate oneness of humanity; they even allow us our conquest over the forces of nature. Yet we do not understand..." (Pg. X, *Insights of a Himalayan Pilgrim.*)

The miracles we had witnessed in the Philippines continued to destabilize what had been the *terra firma* of daily life. Geoff and I had been participants in something beyond our understanding, which pressed us to re-evaluate. It was an experience both blessed and unsettling.

I had felt a new sense of connection to all living things since I was ill, but the magnitude of this connection increased when we visited The Philippines. After Manila the divine bond was also more sustained. I didn't stretch in order to understand it; it wasn't a matter of trying at all, or of needing to go to church to feel transported by it. It was simply there. Shift happens.

Along with this came a myriad of other qualities, which I had previously longed for in my life. There was automatic acceptance, or an ability to see beauty and valor in the full spectrum of fellow-travelers; from the badly burned beggar on the street to the flashy, wealthy ladies in Hong Kong, the tai tais, who very often depended on glitter and wealth to feel alive and worthy. Acceptance replaced a predisposition to be judgmental and critical, not only of others, but also of myself. Trusting in the uniqueness of each individual process, respect and awe of the divine plan replaced the "shoulds." There was no contest.

In addition the strong, sustained feeling of being blessed and loved by Divine Spirit, which Lazaris calls "God/Goddess/All That Is" was marvelous. Whatever name is used, we are all loved and blessed in this way; but most often we don't know how to clear away the static and the blockages in order to tune our spiritual antennae to receive it. Humans wonder: if Divine Spirit doesn't really exist, and we foolishly depend on it, where will we be when the chips are down? Beyond this shibboleth of fear, there is yet another barrier: do we feel worthy enough to receive divine blessings? Some of us feel it would be greedy to consider asking. In this way we ignorantly limit the power of Divine Spirit.

The world I knew best was about egos and the need to be in control. We were all harnessed to ambitious treadmills, reaching to fulfill potential. We wanted to send our children to good schools and excellent colleges, to provide travel and exposure, and to be comfortable in the world. Like hamsters we ran round and round the wheel of accomplishment. In trying to do it better and faster, we became accustomed to the creak of the wheel. Seduced by familiarity, the sound of the treadmill ultimately replaced the richness, the varied dimensions of life itself. There wasn't any time or inclination to develop a living relationship with Divine Spirit or with our higher selves. To activate this relationship there must be time for inner quiet on a daily basis. What I experienced most was noise; from time to time I wondered about it. Wasn't life meant to be richer somehow?

Meditation shuts out the noise, provides a still place, and allows the opening up process. We are presented with the opportunity to become whole rather than scattered, focused instead of rambling, and to receive divine direction. Sogyal Rinpoche, a Tibetan monk and author of *The Tibetan Book of Living and Dying*, explains, "It is only through meditation that you can undertake the journey to discover your true nature, and so find the stability and confidence you will need to live and die well."

For me, choosing to meditate was a life and death issue. This place of inner quiet is where real healing can occur. It is where the body's healing pharmacy opens for business. Finding this place of quiet is one of the singularly most important things we can do for ourselves. It provides us with an arena and an opportunity to make good life choices. The Manila experience was a part of this.

Geoff spent time trying to find a niche in his beautifully constructed Harvard honeycomb of knowledge, a place into which he could file Manila and relate it to something he already knew. Healers have told me that this need to make things fit is an admirable quality; but conversely it creates a tendency to hold the mind closed, obstructing new growth. As a group, men tend to hinge their reality on what is written, provable, measurable, and/or certified. If it hangs on the wall in a black frame with seals and signatures, all the better. Having said this, the men I know who are healers are extremely powerful channels for divine energy.

To a lesser degree, I also looked for a niche where I could put th. new set of experiences, if only to explain it to friends; but feeling preceded thought, and I couldn't feel anything but profoundly blessed when Gary Magno removed the tumor from my body. In realizing that I could never find a known logical framework for these miracles, I skipped over most of the head exercises and reckoned that it was a life-prolonging gift. That was more than enough.

On our last day in Manila I had asked Gary if I should make an appointment to come back in six months time.

"Not now," was his answer. "If you need to come back for healing, you will know it." Then he had added, "You will also know when you are finished with all of this. Your sessions went very well."

I stayed quiet on The Peak for several days. After this short gestation period there was a great urge to tell my family in America. I telephoned Cindy first. She listened carefully and then asked a barrage of challenging and protective questions: "How do you know it wasn't a trick? Did the healer wear a long-sleeved shirt? Did he charge you a fortune?" (He didn't wear a long-sleeved shirt, and he hadn't charged a thing. We made a donation.) "How do you think a human being can do this?"

"I know it sounds too bizarre to be true, but it happened just as I have described it," I answered. "I could feel the blood squirting out."

Cindy concluded that it was a miracle which, like the other miracles, had probably been arranged for me. Oddly enough she especially liked the brass fifty-cent piece, which had dropped as a prelude at the airport. My logical brother-in-law was in awe of the Manila story. He couldn't understand it, but he was able to believe it had really happened.

My mother's reaction was lovely. Having urged us for years to give up the ex-patriots' gypsy life and return to America, she took a deep breath and said, "I'm beginning to realize that you have been in Asia for a reason. It has been an incredible place for you to grow and now to heal. There aren't any accidents, you know. I am so glad that you went to Manila."

Daddy wanted to understand but couldn't. Still his response was, "Whatever works, I am supportive of it, and I am always supportive of you."

Peter wrote an English paper about our time in Manila, causing a stir in the small Massachusetts town where he attended school. A teacher with an ailing father wrote to me for more information, and a few parents wanted to discuss experiences over the telephone.

Other than my family I confided in a handful of special friends. Geoff was much more restrained, having been cautioned by his father, a retired radiologist, to be very circumspect. Given the nature of our society, this well-intended advice probably served Geoff well. It wasn't brave, but it was safe. Within a relatively short period of time, however, Geoff opened up and told his closest friends.

With naiveté and in the interest of sharing information, I decided to revisit the doctor I had seen at The Matilda Hospital. Once again I climbed onto the examining table, and she began to probe the area of concern. This time she couldn't find a trace of the lump. Sitting on the table, I related what had happened in Manila. I opened my handbag and took out a packet of photographs. We had reluctantly hired a photographer ourselves, on the advice of a friend in Hong Kong. ("Be sure to find someone to take unobtrusive photos of the healing session," she had cautioned. "Your family and friends will have a better chance to understand what you went through. Otherwise they might think you have 'gone over the top.'")

The doctor perused the prints in a way which seemed at first to be expressionless. I soon realized that she was controlling her emotions.

"I went to one of the best healers in The Philippines," I told her, "and he removed the tumor that you felt several weeks ago." I said it straight out. "It was the same shape that you described."

There was a frozen moment. Then I continued.

"I should also tell you that I didn't tell the healer anything at all about your examination."

The doctor was both threatened and intrigued by my story.

"I can't believe this," she finally said. "It goes against everything that I have ever learned. My family is made up of scientists, you see."

She looked down at her desk, deliberating over whether or not to soften her remarks.

"I don't think you are lying," she said, "but this is beyond my understanding."

"You should know that it is also beyond mine. I don't know where to put this experience in the scientific world as we know it, but my husband came with me. He watched everything from less than a foot away. It wasn't a magic trick." There was a short pause.

"I came back to see you because I thought that as a medical doctor, and I suppose, as a woman, you would be interested. It seemed to me to be the right thing to do."

In the end, this exasperated doctor found an intellectually comfortable niche. "I think the original lump I felt must have been a piece of poo," she said. Then she began to straighten her already tidy des

I was disappointed and disheartened, remembering anecdotal s
of patients sharing healing information with their doctors.

Responses from close friends, on the other hand, were overwhelm
ingly positive. I showed some of them the photographs and described
what I had seen, heard, and smelled. A few of them were not surprised
at all; the majority was in awe. Most would have gone to Manila themselves, if the need arose. One British friend, Philippa, found it fascinating, but too much of a stretch, in spite of her own experience of cancer.
A short time later Philippa's husband was transferred to Australia, and I
gave her a farewell luncheon.

She invited a small group of CanSurvive friends (a cancer support
group in Hong Kong), who had helped her in an initial bout with breast
cancer nearly five years before. At lunch I was asked to recount the
Manila experience. I did. Reluctantly I showed the photographs as well.
By the end of the luncheon I had agreed to receive screened calls from
likely candidates for psychic healing on the CanSurvive Hot Line. It is this
connection which leads to the next part of my story.

A few weeks later, an Englishman, Chris, telephoned late one afternoon. He had benign tumors in his lungs, which were theoretically dou-
bling in size each year. He had heard about the healers in The Philippines
and specifically about my experience with Gary Magno.

"Who recommended him? What does the healer actually do? Could
you feel anything?" And then the ultimate question, "Did Gary Magno
wear a long-sleeved shirt?"

I told him that he hadn't. "But you have brought up a very important
point. If you decide to go to a healer in The Philippines, be sure that you
see a legitimate one. Don't go to anyone without a firsthand recommendation. It is also important that the recommendation be current.
Occasionally the good healers become ensnarled in commercial ventures
and as a consequence lose their abilities. Many of them are frauds who
mess about with animal parts. My friends in Manila have warned me. Do
be careful. It is an extremely poor country. People do desperate things
for money."

"I would like to give you something in return for your help," Chris
said, "or perhaps I should say someone. There is an amazing lady called
Rosemary Altea here. She is a medium and a healer visiting from the UK."

"Have you seen her already?"

"Oh yes. She has helped me. Try to see her if you can. She is a phenomenal medium."

I said thank you and we said good-bye, agreeing to actually meet me. I hung up the telephone, and in the silence reckoned that I recently taken too many giant steps in this "phenomenal" world. ere hadn't been enough time to assimilate the experience so far.

And how many of "these people" did I need to know, anyway?

15

Every time it rains, it rains pennies from heaven...

—Irving Berlin

The number three had become significant in my life. If something I was considering came up three times, it was an indication that I should follow through. I have since learned that this number is significant for many, many people.

In the next 24 hours, Rosemary Altea's name came up twice again, and I soon found myself at a very small dinner party in her honor. There were about ten of us, all women, eating informally from plates on our laps. The dinner had been organized by one of the guests at Philippa's luncheon. We chatted as women do; then Rosemary told us about herself.

For as long as she could remember she had heard voices and seen spirit beings. Her family in England had discouraged her from talking about these experiences and threatened to send her to "The Tower," a place to which Rosemary's grandmother had been committed from time to time. (Grandmother had also heard voices, seen spirit beings, and thought herself to be crazy.)

Still the spirits seemed to gather around Rosemary, hoping to have a chance to speak. Rosemary has a Spirit Guide called Grey Eagle, an Apache Shaman, who lived long ago. (There is a photograph of Grey Eagle in Robert Utley's book, *The Lance and the Shield*.)

"Grey Eagle is wonderful," she said, "my dearest friend in all the world. But before he came to me I resisted the very thought of having a Red Indian Spirit Guide. It seemed too much of a fashion. Everyone claims to have either an Indian guide, a hooded old sage, or a nun. I didn't want any of these. But then we don't have choices about these things."

81

remember asking Rosemary if she shared Grey Eagle with others. "No," she said, "he works just with me."

(In a meditation a few weeks earlier, I too, had seen an Indian. He was tall and brave looking, with a no-nonsense expression on his face. I respected him and liked the way he looked. In this particular meditation he was standing next to Nana, who was wearing her blue dress.

"What is your name?" I had asked.

"Red Feather," he answered.

I had rolled my eyes and thought, "*Red Feather?* Gimme a break." Then I opened my eyes and thought it was all a silly play of the imagination.)

"Don't some of the shaman guides move around among a small group of people?" I asked Rosemary.

"No," she answered, then pausing as though she was trying to think this through, she continued. "There is one who does, though. He goes to sick people, makes his rounds like a doctor or a healer would, and once they are well, he moves on."

"Does he have a name?"

"Red Feather," was her answer.

"Red Feather!" I affirmed incredulously.

"Yes. Have you heard of him?" she asked.

"Well, sort of."

Near the end of the evening Rosemary spoke to a young woman who sat directly across from her on the sofa.

"There is a sweet little girl just behind you," she said. "She has curly blonde hair and blue eyes, and she is wearing a pretty summer dress, a sundress with little straps crossed at the back."

The woman began to cry.

"She is your daughter, isn't she?" Rosemary asked very gently.

The woman was visibly overtaken. She explained that her daughter had died quite suddenly two years before.

"She is lovely and full of energy," Rosemary went on. "She wants me to tell you that she is absolutely fine and that she is near you all of the time. She is smiling now."

The woman took a kleenex from her handbag and wiped her eyes. We all did.

"She asks me to tell you that she is worried about one of your large plants. Does that make sense to you?"

The woman replied immediately. "No, it doesn't. I have no idea what you mean."

"All right, then let me try this another way," Rosemary went on. She was quiet for a few moments, characteristically looking down towa. floor, as though the answer would be there. "Your daughter tells me the plant is really big. It is growing outside in the garden, and it has fa en down. It needs a stake to hold it up."

The woman, suddenly bursting with pride and enthusiasm said, "Yes, of course! Of course! She is quite right. One of the really tall bushes in the garden blew over in the typhoon last week, and I haven't tended to it."

We were all awestruck. The living room was absolutely silent. It was inspirational.

Rosemary soon included the rest of us in the conversation.

"This is the kind of evidence you should expect from a good medium," she said. "It tells you that she or he is really in touch with the other side."

Having established that, Rosemary went on to tell more.

"I never use the word 'died.' I usually say 'passed over.' It is much more precise. I don't consider the people I see and speak to to be dead. They are very much alive. It's just that the rest of you can't see them."

Rosemary had come to Hong Kong for a month at the invitation of friends the year before. She quickly developed a loyal following. Clients established in Hong Kong would often telephone her in the UK when they needed help. She gave sittings to clients during the day, for which she charged a reasonable fee. In the evenings she gave healing to those who needed it. Remuneration for this was entirely on a donation basis. Rosemary has several small, non-profit healing centres in the North of England, staffed with other experienced healers.

Her problem in Hong Kong was that she didn't have a place to work. She had explored the possibility of using a hotel room on a daily basis, but it was too expensive. Someone suggested a small space adjoining an office, but that would have been disruptive with telephones ringing, fax machines beeping and foot traffic.

I telephoned Rosemary the day after the little dinner party and offered the use of our house for healing sessions. "I was thinking that you could do one session in the morning and another in the evening," I offered.

"It sounds lovely," she said. "Thank you very much."

We went on to discuss dates and getting maps to people who wanted to come.

"For the day session," I continued, "why don't you stay for a simple lunch? We'll have a couple of chicken tetrazzini casseroles and a salad, French bread, something easy, for anyone who wants to stay."

hat sounds great."

t was a worthwhile and rich experience. After the first healing ses-
n, we all moved into the living room where Rosemary described all
orts of details from pet names, to the style of a crocheted toilet paper
cover one patient's English grandmother had made when he was a small
child.

Rosemary had also warned someone about buying a property in
Canada the year before.

"There are problems with water," she had said. "The property is
beautiful but very risky."

The man took her advice to the extent of having the house and property carefully checked out. Not finding a problem anywhere, he decided
to go ahead with the purchase. Within six months of closing the deal,
there was an unusually heavy rainfall. The hillside slid onto one wing of
the house, completely destroying it. The gentleman came and told his
story.

"The problem was insufficient drainage off the hill." He then stated
the obvious. "I had no way of knowing this would happen, but I have a
real headache now."

The following day was quieter, but equally interesting. A couple of
concerned wives brought their husbands in for healing, virtually sneak-
ing them up from the Financial District, fortunately at different times.
They would come in only if I swore not to tell any of our mutual friends,
or mention their visits to my husband. One managing director was a
chain-smoker, whose wife adored him and worried about his health.

After the healing about eleven stayed for lunch. Rosemary was pre-
dictably fascinating. My dear friend, who had sent me to the medium in
Massachusetts two years before, happened to be visiting with her husband for our 25th wedding anniversary party. After lunch, we lingered
over coffee and fruit and cookies. Rosemary sat at one end of the table;
I was at the other.

This time she addressed me.

"Would you like to know who is standing just behind you?" she
asked.

I instinctively glanced over my right shoulder. Not seeing anyone, I
answered, "No. No, I wouldn't, at least not now." Then I added, "Could
you tell me later?"

"I might," she said.

But the seeds of curiosity had been sprinkled and the table came
alive with voices wanting to know.

"Come on, tell us. Who is there?"

My curiosity was baited, too, and in spite of a wish for privacy, I ___ in.

"All right, Rosemary."

Rosemary dragged her feet a little and feigned refusal. Then she conceded.

"There is a sweet older lady with gray curly hair. She is wearing a blue dress and an apron."

A blue dress.

Rosemary continued. "The apron is quite funny. It looks like a piece of white linen, which has been fed onto a white plastic hoop. It loops around the waist like an oversized headband."

"Amazing," I said. "I had forgotten all about that apron. I haven't seen it for ages, 25 years or more. And the blue dress. They both belong to my Swedish grandmother."

"Well she looks ridiculous! Your grandmother is laughing now because I am telling you how funny she looks. She looks comical because of the deep pockets in the apron."

"I remember those, too," I said. "She always kept white linen handkerchiefs in them."

Rosemary continued. "The pockets are like old-fashioned shoe caddies, the kind people used to hang on the back of closet doors. Well these pockets are absolutely bulging! They are pulling on the apron, weighing it down. She actually does look very funny." Rosemary laughed. She was really enjoying herself now.

"Why are they bulging?" I asked.

"Hold on," Rosemary said. "Let me have a look."

She looked askance at the floor in a way that I had come to know. Then she said, "Pennies. Pennies. Does that mean anything to you?"

"Yes," I nodded, unable to speak. It was hard to believe.

"Your grandmother tells me that you have been finding a lot of them. You have thought the pennies are for luck. They aren't. She wants you to know that the pennies are for hope. She also wants me to tell you that she is determined to help you, to show you how to make your way out of this disease and back to health. She will show you things in the realm of healing that she didn't know about in time for her own recovery. She tells me that she has shown you some already."

More tears and smiling, I could only nod. No one spoke or made a sound for a long time. When I finally looked up, there was a box of Kleenex circling around the table.

16

Gud som haver barnen kär
Se till mig om liten är
Vart jag mig I världen vandrer
Står min lycka I Guds händer.

—Traditional Swedish Children's Prayer

God, who holds the children dear,
Look after me, for I am small.
Wherever I wander in the world
My happiness is in your hands.

—English translation

Even though Nana had passed on several years before, she had been such an exceptional presence that memories of her, and the positive, loving influence she exuded were very much a part of me. Still, on a daily basis, I had had a rather milder sense of her being. From a dimension so rich in kindness, it was an especially desirable place. I remembered vividly once again how she looked, the scent of her daphne perfume, and her kitchen, faintly scented with apples. I could see her in the mornings, turning on the gas furnace in the dining room fireplace to warm the house. Not knowing what else to do, I spoke to her with my heart, appreciative of the best memories of childhood, and understandably overflowing with thanks for what she was doing to help me now. With Nana's patient willingness to illuminate my journey, there was a feeling of being enveloped in a blanket of pink cashmere love. It was clear that she was a tenacious presence. She would support and protect me with all she was worth, a distinctly clear advantage. It was clear that I was still in a difficult spot, but she was, without doubt, helping steer the course. It was a feeling that is hard to describe.

For days, perhaps weeks after the luncheon party I retraced all penny incidents and spent a good deal of time reflecting on what I learned and been shown.

Walking many times around The Peak, it was easy to remember how splendidly the coins had been delivered, with humor, with great precision, surprise and timeliness. Thanks to dear Rosemary I had found another world, another explanation, which was enormously beneficial. It is probable that in the spirit of hope and the expectation of positive results, I owe my life to it.

I knew the most that doctors, healers, drugs, remedies, machines and methods can do is to assist our bodies in healing. At the very least the large initial task we have to accomplish is to free ourselves from negative thoughts, from patterns in life which harm us, and from limiting expectations, which hold us hostage. This is an enormous undertaking, vitally empowering for the healer *within*. Of course, doctors can set bones, stitch cuts, give injections and remove unwanted matter. While these procedures can be life saving, it is the healer within which must be engaged, connected with the divine, and supported, to achieve the best possible result.

And what about personal qualities? I had always had an open, though conservatively-paced attitude and outlook. There was a willingness to explore and take considered chances, to look for the unique, sometimes scary truth and to go beyond the interests of "the experts," because I knew that invariably there is always more to know. From the very beginning it was clear that no one could simply deliver me to a state of wellness. It doesn't work that way. The allopathic medical experts, thank heaven, knew enough to help me buy the time in which to find my way, and for that I was and am extremely grateful. Without them I wouldn't be here; had I depended solely on their approach, I wouldn't be here, either. Could Nana have influenced the expanded approach to healing which I had sought out? Was she similar to a Guardian Angel? Or more like a spokesman on my behalf in another realm?

How many times had the clues that were put before me been missed? How many times had I fallen into the black pit of fear? And what about the days of going backward, of being lost entirely? The times, which culminated with an angry cry in the field of screaming cicadas, "Who is in charge here? Where are you? I want to see the manager, please."

On these occasions, down in the dark, hopeless places, petrified by fear, I felt like a champagne cork, bobbing in a giant sea. I desperately didn't want to leave my children. I couldn't leave them. By going into and *through* these feelings of utter despair, it was possible to sort out the dark s and to come back into the healing realm. Who helped?

From time to time many of us sense the closeness of someone we ve who has died; they are in the car, at the wedding, or present at nother special occasion. Sometimes there is a dream in which these loved ones speak to us, or laugh, offering important insights.

Nana's pennies were a similar presence; they absolutely carried me away, and still do. I wanted to hold her for a very long time without saying anything and to feel her next to me. I wanted to cry with her and to say out loud, with all of my heart, "Thank you. You were and you are my special one."

She had always encouraged the embracing of the unknown and sparkled with the adventure of it. From this time and in this new realm I began to think of my Swedish grandmother as Nana Bluedress.

It was also in this period that I found a remarkable oncologist whom I could trust. His name is Dr. William Buchholz.

While pursuing an uncharted course, I knew it would be important to find a proficient medical doctor who could monitor progress. It wasn't that I didn't trust what I was doing; it was necessary and sensible to confirm where my body was in the process. In Bill Buchholz I found this and much more.

With the exception of Bernie Siegel and Carl Simonton (neither of whom I had met), oncologists seemed to me to be a curious group of individuals. Is it because they are so burdened by the misery and suffering of their patients that they often seem to be removed and lacking warmth? Are they afraid of becoming too attached or consumed by the situations of people in their care? They seem to place whatever trust they have in the chemotherapy recipe and give very little credence to innate healing possibilities. When cancer patients do heal, a dreadful term is used by the traditional medical world to define it: "spontaneous remission." The word seems to say, "You are living with a loaded gun which, at the moment, isn't firing for some mysterious reason, but it could go off at any time. Any time." The phrase comes with an implicit charge to anticipate a blow. In our litigious society would it be too risky to say, "You are progressing beautifully in the healing process; keep up the good work," and leave it there?

The scientific method has, to a large extent, displaced touch, prayer, and the healing power of words and feelings. Machinery provides test results, gathers statistics and controls our world. In my healing world, odds and probabilities define a very limited reality. Science is a god, and doctors, often referred to as demi-gods, have their own particular truth. Patients who blindly embrace this paradigm are taking a great risk. They abdicate personal responsibility and accept the unspoken notion that metaphorically they have more in common with a late model car than with being human. The doctors I am close to are aware of the powerful energy which can be activated to accomplish wellness; they are not demigods, but at this time they are unusual. I love and admire them, recognizing that they embody the blessed combination.

One oncologist tried to cheer me up when I was initially diagnosed. "Don't worry, we've kept one patient with your kind of cancer going for twelve years!"

I thought to myself, I'm living to be ninety at least, and I'm not depending entirely on you to get me there, but I am grateful that you are helping me.

I also had the unfortunate experience of listening to an oncologist let off steam at a large dinner party in Boston. He had no idea of my health history and was too absorbed in what he was saying to notice that I was wearing a wig. He started the conversation by proudly telling me that he was affiliated with one of America's finest private clinics. (It was a clinic I had abstracted medical records from; this evaluation was correct.)

He then went on to say, "I'm so glad when Saturdays come and I am not on call."

"Being on call must be one of the difficult aspects of what you do."

"No, the difficult part is being with those horrible sick people all week! I am so glad to be away from them."

Had this happened to me now I would have probably said, "I can imagine that it must be hard. I have often wondered about that. I don't know how my oncologist does it. You have a very difficult profession." But at the time it was such a jarring thing to hear, I wanted to hit him without mercy, pull off my wig and ask, "Why don't you consider another line of work if this is too much for you?"

Instead I turned and walked away, leaving it to the grapevine.

Thank heaven for Bill Buchholz. With Dr. Buchholz I have been able to combine sensible traditional medicine with my own healing course. When we initially met, in 1989, he was wearing a white lab coat with a tiny gold angel on the lapel, something far less common then than now. There was a sign in his office describing the value of hugs, and he gives real ones. Reprints of his article from *The Journal of the American Medical Association* described a very special over-the-counter remedy: *A Prescription for Hope*, which is referenced in the Highly Recommended Books list. He had also framed the Chinese character for Crisis with its definition: DANGER AND OPPORTUNITY.

Bill's first words to me were, "Tell me what I can do to support you .n your healing," and we took it from there.

I asked him to monitor my progress; then I asked for his patience, explaining that I was following an unusual course. His official position, we agreed, would be Keeper of the Films. His presence sought to keep me connected with respect to the allopathic medical world, which he believed to be vital to my survival.

The exam was fine, and within days I was winging my way back to Hong Kong, wondering if I hadn't turned the corner on this dreadful disease. It seemed nearly over. Nearly.

17

At some level, all things are interconnected...we are all part of one another. Thoughts influence all living things...If people become aware of this they will have a far greater respect for one another and a far greater respect for the environment. That, in itself, is a form of healing as far as I am concerned.

—Matthew Manning

Within a month of returning to Hong Kong, my English friend, Chris, telephoned to say that he had gone to see a preeminent healer in the South of England. His name was Matthew Manning. With the passing of Harry Edwards, Matthew is often referred to as Britain's greatest healer. The most exciting scoop was that Matthew would be coming to Hong Kong in a month's time to give one of his healing seminars. Chris urged me to sign on right away.

Matthew's work in the area of healing and teaching are well worth describing. Of all the healers I had been blessed to know, Matthew had, up to that time, taught me the most about wellness. In claiming for ourselves the components of a healthy life, we often have the opportunity to move toward deactivating disease in our physical bodies.

When Matthew was young, he spent a brief period as a "metal bender," much in the style of Uri Geller. Matthew would go on British television before a live audience and bend forks, keys, anything metal, using his mental concentration. In very little time he became a celebrity of sorts. Eventually he found that this was an approach to life which left him feeling quite empty. His performances gave rise to sensationalism and commercialism, and he soon discovered this was an extremely unsatisfying way in which to live. He wanted to use his unique powers in a more creative, contributory way.

Following a personal experience of enlightenment in Northern India, ..e was led to become a healer. His work has since been studied in var-..ous countries, including not only the U.K., but also the United States, Canada, and Sweden. He has worked with research scientists and met with Nobel Prize winners, participating in experiments designed to show the effects of his brain waves on plants and seeds, gerbils, fish and human beings.

It was through one of these experiments in Canada that it became known that Matthew's brain waves are unique; their patterns had never been seen or recorded by scientists before. When he was focusing on a subject, patterns were emitted from the hypothalamus, or old brain. This part of the brain is thought to be inactive, though prehistoric man used it extensively.

It is Matthew's belief that we are all capable of using this area of the brain, but that it has atrophied for lack of use. Intuition lodges there, as do psychic powers. Nearing the end of the 20th Century we no longer have the need to look within, as, for example, the Aboriginal people do, to survive. We have created a society in which everything is provided for us. It isn't necessary for us to know the direction in which to find food, water, or shelter from a storm. We depend on telephones, faxes, computers and filofaxes, experts and machines to tell us whatever we need or want, and then where to find it.

When I first met Matthew, he spent the majority of his time helping people from all over the world in his healing room in Suffolk. He is a particularly fine and fascinating teacher, as well, sharing generously all that he knows. He tells us that we are our own best healers; we need only to realize it. He believes that there are three invaluable ingredients in the healing process:

DESIRE (to be well)

BELIEF (that one can get well), and most importantly (as this aspect is most often left out)

EXPECTATION (that one is actually getting well)

This group of words was familiar. Many people can manifest desire and belief; but they either forget to include expectation, or undervalue it, or sense it intermittently.

As we analyze these ingredients in our lives, the mix is more complicated than it appears. We might think we have a desire to be well, but is it really so? What we might actually intend on a deeper level is to leave this life. Perhaps we have suffered a great loss (loss of a loved one, a job,

or perhaps of attention). Maybe we have been betrayed; sometimes w
are boxed into a marriage we dislike but can't see a clear way out of.
Peculiar as it sounds, death can serve as the ultimate clean divorce, a
clean exit. There is a certain amount of detective work involved in dis-
covering what we really desire.

The main tools Matthew encourages us to use are relaxation and
visualization. It is in the state of relaxed meditation that our brains produce alpha waves, the same waves that occur naturally when we sleep.
Alpha waves neutralize stress, providing the physical bodies with a cli-
mate in which optimum healing can occur.

Matthew directs us, as Reiki Masters do, to clean up daily language,
to be aware of such phrases as, "This job is killing me." "He is a pain in
the neck or the ass." "It makes me sick to think about it."

He also encourages us to engage more than one healer if we feel we
need to. He admits that he cannot help everyone, and that he has more
success with some diseases than with others. Matthew believes in the
value of orthodox medicine, viewing his work as complimentary to it. In
England there is a developing tradition of cooperation between registered healers and the medical profession. Healers are allowed into hos-
pitals to treat their patients. Ironically, it is the English clergy, not the doctors, who have been the most resistant to this approach.

Matthew believes that while no one knows the real dynamics of healing, what he and other healers accomplish is to give the physical body a
"boost." The individual can then carry on with his or her own healing
from there. The potential of this "boost" is described in the following
experiment carried out in 1977, in San Antonio, Texas. Quoted with
Matthew's permission, he writes:

"This was an experiment which I did with Dr. John Kemmetz, and
which, to my mind, has the most vital implications for medicine and healing. For many, many years there have been healers who have been able
to help cancer patients. There are many cancer patients, who, because of
the intervention of a healer, have had a remission of their disease, or who
have improved considerably.

"The reaction from orthodox doctors is invariably the same. They will
usually say that patients might have got well, anyway. Sometimes they
will say that it was just faith, that because the person believed they were
going to be healed that that, in itself, healed them.

"I had been doing this experiment in San Antonio working with cervical cancer cells, grown in plastic flasks. They grow across the bottom
of the flask in a kind of layer of carpet. These cells stick to the inside of
the container with an electrostatic charge. It is the same kind of charge

ou get if you run a balloon up and down your front; you can then stick t to the wall.

"There is nothing which apparently will cause these cells to break free naturally from the inside of the container. They have been shaken, they have been heated, they have been frozen, they have been dropped.

"The only time the cancer cell breaks free is if for any reason its metabolism is charged, if the cell is injured, or if the cell dies. At that point the electrostatic charge on the surface of the cell is broken, and it falls into the solution of liquid protein.

"Now the cancer cells are dying and regenerating all of the time. Being cancer cells, they regenerate much faster than they die. Each cell keeps reproducing like crazy. They do this naturally. And when the cells die, then obviously they break free from the inside of the container and they start to float around in this pink liquid protein.

"Before the experiment begins, we put the liquid under a microscope and count the number of dead cancer cells per milliliter of liquid; in other words we can count the cells that have died through natural circumstances.

"Next I am given one of the plastic containers to hold in my hands for twenty minutes. Another container is given to somebody else who does not claim to have healing abilities, and they try to imitate whatever I do. A third flask is just left on a bench top and nobody touches it at all.

"I then imagine that I am surrounding the whole container with white light. I have seen the cells under a microscope, so I know what they look like. I imagine that I am surrounding every single cell with white light. And then I just imagine that mentally I am talking to the cancer cells. I tell them that their use on this level of reality is finished and they have to go somewhere else.

"After twenty minutes of healing, the container is opened by Dr. Kemmetz. Another sample of the liquid is removed, and he counts the number of dead cells again.

"We'd got results 27 times out of 30 that we'd done the experiment. Those containers held by someone else or left on the bench top had never registered any difference. However, the containers which I had been holding (which I had been healing), had enormous differences in the number of dead cells.

"After twenty minutes of healing, the number of dead cells usually increased from 200% to 1200%. It is very, very difficult to explain results like that simply in terms of natural remissions. Cancer cells in plastic flasks, to the best of my knowledge, do not have natural remissions."

"The cancer cells were actually being killed by Matthew," Dr.

Kemmetz commented after the experiment. "Once they had br.
away, they were not viable cells any longer. In at least 60% of the ca:
the results were quite significant. When an individual who is not
Psychic Healer tried to do the same thing, we didn't get anything."

Dr. William Braud, who was also involved in the experiments, concluded, "Matthew has demonstrated that he can influence cancer cells.
There may be parapsychological factors involved that could be used to
heal others. It is a valid avenue for us to explore."

Matthew Manning is an extraordinary healer. He was enormously
helpful in bringing all of my healing experiences into a clearer focus, to
affirm the invaluable threads of belief I had begun to weave into something more substantial. He helped me to synthesize and further understand the story so far. It was definitely a hero's journey. But it wasn't over
yet.

18

It is important to recognize that 'scientific reality' is methodologically limited to physical reality.

—Mary Scott

Within six weeks of Matthew's Hong Kong seminar I discovered another lump in my abdomen. It was a terrible blow, calling to task once again the unorthodox approach to healing I had taken. After two or three weeks of living with this discovery, it was verified by a C-T Scan at the Seventh Day Adventist Hospital in Hong Kong. The Chinese American radiologist in charge had practiced medicine previously in Napa, California. On reviewing the new films, his soft and gentle manner became grave.

The disease was classified as "active." After all I had been through, how could it be? The doctor gave me a list of local oncologists and offered to make introductions. I was genuinely appreciative but told him that I had some thinking to do.

We left the hospital, and after a little quiet time together, Geoff went back to the office and I went home to our terrace overlooking The South China Sea, a quiet place from which to ask what to do. Neither Geoff nor I knew if we were moving toward yet another hard patch or some kind of resolution. Disaster seemed to be in the lead, and I was devastated inside. It was a demoralizing time, two steps forward, one step back at best.

By now the process of asking for guidance had become almost second nature to me. By sitting quietly in a relaxed place, free of disturbance, I knew where to go to make the connection. I would cleanse myself by imagining an old-fashioned toilet lever at the top of my head. With one pull on the chain, the color blue would run down through me and out of the bottom of my feet, flowing deeply into the center of the

96

Earth. Rosemary had taught me this. Soon after I would take a few deep breaths with exuberant exhalings and go deeper into the stillness. It was there that I asked for direction. Given this new turn of events with the C-T Scan, what was the best course to follow? In both the asking and the listening I surrendered any need to control the outcome. Answers always came, sometimes immediately; more often they came within three days or so.

Common sense had told me it would be counterproductive to initiate yet another relationship with an oncologist in Hong Kong. I already had an excellent doctor in California. But there were other choices. For a start I could easily fly to Manila to see Gary Magno, or I could try to get an appointment with Matthew Manning in England. There could be significant waiting periods in both cases, but I could try.

The answer was given to me clearly, but in a way that is difficult to explain. Two days later, as I walked around Lugard Road on The Peak, it was simply there, in my consciousness, announced without words, and strongly. There was not an alternative, no Plan B, and it was definitely not conjured up. I didn't agree with the direction. I was told to go and see Dr. Buchholz in Mountain View, California. Why? It didn't make logical sense. Visiting either of the healers seemed a far more practical idea. In short I couldn't understand the answer, but having begun to have an idea of how these sorts of things work, I trusted the message.

Within a few days, making my way across the Pacific, the answer was still puzzling. This was not the obvious solution. Was this the right course of action?

Two days after my arrival, Cindy and I were in Bill's office. He reviewed the films, commented on their technical excellence, and verified the Hong Kong diagnosis. There was indeed a malignant tumor. But for me there was far less fear around it.

While probing and pressing, Bill remarked on its peculiar shape.

"What is different about it?" I asked with some trepidation.

"It seems to be flat rather than rounded, as most of these types of tumors are," he mused. "Curious."

(Before leaving Hong Kong a very fine healer and Reiki Master had been giving me healing massages twice a week. After several sessions, she felt that the lump was beginning to dissolve, and had smiled as she mentioned its "flattening shape" to me.)

In this meeting with Bill Buchholz I didn't feel as petrified as I had been with the Hong Kong radiologist, but it was terribly discouraging and demoralizing. Whatever had been the point of any of this?

It seemed to me that I had followed the healing course, which had

.n presented to me; I had done it with increasing amounts of faith and ...ist. My loved ones supported me, at times with crossed fingers behind .heir backs, hoping, hoping that I was on a legitimate track. Other times I knew they were silently humming the melody from "The Twilight Zone" television program, wondering what I would come up with next.

Finally even I began to have doubts. How could I have followed such a bizarre program? If the alternatives I had chosen were really valid, why didn't the experts in the medical world study them? I knew of doctors who had visited healers and had had good results. Why did they remain anonymous? Does healing run the risk of reversing itself under the negative scrutiny of others? Had my healing been reversed for some reason? Wasn't this all a pretty risky, tenuous business? And, after all I had gone through, why was there a tumor on my report card? Where were the high marks for listening and responding? We seemed to be back at the beginning and while there was less fear, there was angry confusion, as I cried inside with hopelessness. I didn't fully understand that healing is an ongoing process.

After looking at the films once more, and examining me thoroughly, Dr. Buchholz addressed me in a very serious way. His tone softened, but had a clear professional punch.

"I would like to start you on a regime of chemotherapy right away."

Zap. Sucked into the doomsday place, off to the fearful pit I went, before the sentence was completed. I had been seriously betrayed. In a flash, the entire healing course was invalidated, as a figment of foolish imagination, not to mention the poor judgment and stupidity.

Then my voice came back, and I answered in a slow trickle of words, paced carefully, so as not to cry.

"You know, Bill, I don't think I could go through that again."

The first treatment in September, 1998 flashed back in its full intensity. The chemicals had arrived nearly four hours late, as Cindy and I sat on the side of the hospital bed in terrified anticipation. The pharmacy was especially busy, the nurses had explained several times. The prescription would, no doubt, be coming soon.

After more than three and a half-hours of waiting, I had telephoned Bob Albo. With the surgical aspect of my treatment completed, he was technically no longer part of the medical team, but he was the only good friend I could turn to. I told him that I was going to leave the hospital and why. Waiting for nearly four hours in fear was the most patently inhumane and stressful situation I had ever found myself in; how could anyone respect a system like this? Or the hospital?

How could we be talking about healing here? This couldn't be good

for me. What harmful drugs was my body's pharmacy producing
fear and waiting?

Bob was outraged and I was glad. He asked me to hang on for
teen minutes more. Just fifteen minutes. Magically, within ten minutes the
red-colored chemicals were delivered, and I reluctantly changed into a
flimsy generic hospital gown.

Back in Bill Buchholz's office again in 1990, I said, "I won't go back
for additional chemotherapy treatments. I can't do it."

His voice was calm, reassuring, and surprised.

"No, no. The chemotherapy I have in mind is not what you are think-
ing of."

Breathing again.

"I would prescribe oral tablets," he said, "to be taken over a fairly
short period of time."

Before he had finished the sentence the angels got a blanket apolo-
gy, an emotional "U" turn, and we were off again.

"But," Bill continued, "if we do this, I will want you to be here, in the
Bay Area, not in Hong Kong. We can't do it long distance. I will want to
be the one who is responsible for monitoring you."

By now all component parts, voice, heart, mind, and body, had
reassembled, returning to the room and to the conversation.

"If I were your wife, what would you recommend?" I asked him.

"I would advise you that this terrible disease is making a feeble
attempt to reassert itself. I would urge you to take the chemotherapy
drugs, to seize the opportunity to wipe the cancer out." And then he
added, "This is your chance."

So it was not such a negative report. My situation was less than ideal,
but it was not a complete reversal. The words "feeble aspect of the dis-
ease" meant a lot.

"How much time do I have to decide without putting myself at risk?

Bill said, "Wait until summer, if you want."

"Thank you," I said. "I value your advice." Then there was a pause.
"I would like to consider a couple of other approaches."

"All right," Bill said, and then he gave me a wonderfully refreshing
surprise.

"I will support you in whatever you want to do."

"I will come back to see you in early June," I promised, "just before
my birthday. How does that sound?"

We hugged and said good-bye.

Soon I was flying back to Hong Kong, again listening for feedback
and direction. Where was *this* episode going and what was it about?

full week later, again while walking around The Peak, I decided to
to Geoff about flying to England. The thought came again and again.
was somehow clear that the next step would be to see Matthew
anning. It would not be possible for Geoff to get away, I knew that, but
I could ask Cindy to meet me in London.

"If it takes six months to get an appointment," I remember saying at
dinner, "this plan won't work. I have a follow-up appointment with Bill
Buchholz on the 2nd of June."

Geoff agreed. "Of course we could go back to Gary Magno in
Manila," he mused.

"I know. This was my first idea, too. It would be less expensive
because Gary is closer, and I know he is good, but I think that I am
meant to see Matthew. I feel that participating in his seminar was a preliminary part of this. I am being nudged in this direction."

Geoff was generously supportive; "princely" would be a better word.

"What if Cindy can't get away?" he asked.

"Then I don't think I will go, unless you can somehow come with
me. It would be awful to go alone."

Late that evening I telephoned Cindy in California. She thought it was
an excellent plan. She would see if she could get away; and within the
next two days she arranged it. If I could get the appointments within the
time agreed upon, we would meet in London.

I faxed Matthew's office, telling him about the rough spot that I was
in, asking if I could come to Suffolk for healing. Forty-eight hours later I
had an answer. I would be given a series of ten sessions in two weeks'
time.

Cindy and I met at Heathrow Airport, where Matthew's secretary had
kindly arranged for a car to pick us up. We made our way to the splendid old guild town of Lavenham and tucked in at a 14th Century Inn
called The Swan. Things mysteriously fall into place when a plan is right.

19

Each day is a journey and the journey itself, home.

—Basho, 1689

After checking into The Swan we had a rest, and then had afternoon tea in the lounge by a smoky wood fire. Later we explored the gentle English countryside in search of the Village of Hartest, where Matthew's home and healing room are located.

It was a treat to be together. Once ordinary sisters, with heavy family baggage in our relationship, we had become closest friends. In spite of travel fatigue, we were like the frisky lambs that frolicked nearby over rolling green hillocks. And I quite liked seeing Matthew's home. His wife and children were returning from the day's marketing, and a small barnyard of animals gathered together at the back of the house.

Once we got down to work, the healing sessions were all very similar. Matthew and I sat on canvas-backed director's chairs. Facing me sideways, he placed his right hand on my shoulder and his left hand just left of the solar plexus. This is where the original tumors had been removed and where the new one was trying to claim territory. I had never mentioned the precise location of the tumor; Matthew's hand went immediately to it. It was in this position that he worked for the better part of each hour.

Music played in the background; sounds of the Earth, a whale song in duet with a lyrical flute enhanced the feeling of serenity in the room.

My part in the assignment was simple: to be still and relax. I simply closed my eyes and received the divine healing energy which Matthew channeled.

Over the course of the week, there was a great deal of heat emanating from his hands; I saw blocks of color again: periwinkle blue,

...enta, and purple. Very often there was the sensation of gentle ...ctrical currents passing through me.

After each appointment I was noticeably energized, as though I had ingested megadoses of vitamins and pycnogenol. Once returning to the car, I smiled in irony at my sister, who would be dozing with a book, groggy and in need of a good cup of English tea. I, on the other hand, felt ready to go dancing. I grew less and less heavy in spirit as we moved through the week, and with the lightness came feelings of joy and tremendous relief.

Matthew is a wonderful, phenomenal healer, with a beautiful and intelligent way about him. He had often told us in the Hong Kong seminar, "Remember to be glad you are alive. It is important not to take it for granted."

It was such a pleasant week. Cindy and I were quite sad when it was over. After thanks and farewells, we were driven back to London. Cindy and I then flew our separate ways, both breathing easier.

The appointment with Bill Buchholz was scheduled for June 2nd, the day before my 50th Birthday and family celebrations. Cindy and I were there on the appointed day; I was feeling surprisingly relaxed and comfortable, at full attention, but not at all anxious.

In the examining room we talked together for a little while, as before, about basic bodily functions. Then Dr. Buchholz weighed me and motioned me onto the examining table. He examined lymph glands and checked breasts; then he probed and measured the tumor area, scrutinized his notes, and probed some more.

When the exam was complete, I did up my clothes and Bill went back to his chair and sat down.

"I don't know what you have been doing," he said, scratching his head, "but the tumor has shrunk considerably."

"I am so glad."

He looked up and smiled. "I wouldn't give you chemotherapy if you begged me for it."

There was still something there, but it seemed to be residual. Dr. Buchholz smiled.

"I would like to see you in six months for a C-T Scan."

"Can we talk about it then?" I asked.

"All right. I would *like* you to have a scan then, but we'll talk about it."

There was a fond farewell and we were off to celebrate, nearly skipping down the stairs like a couple of schoolgirls.

As agreed, in six months time, Cindy and I were in Dr. Buchholz's office again. I answered all of his pertinent questions, feeling more itive than ever, and predisposed to a good result.

Dr. Buchholz weighed me and again motioned me onto the exam ing table, where, as before, he probed my abdominal area with his ma: terful fingers.

After that he made a few notes, then looked up with a sunbeam smile on his face.

"I remember that the last year around this time when you were here, I suggested chemotherapy and you politely declined. You had other directions, which you wanted to follow."

I nodded.

"And when you were here six months ago, we agreed to discuss the C-T Scan I wanted you to have today."

I nodded again.

"I am so proud of you," he said, "for following your own brave independent course. You have done a beautiful job of healing yourself." Then he paused and added, "You won't need a C-T Scan this year."

It was as though I was suddenly alone in the room, transported to a place of silence and buoyant brightness. Here was an electric joy, quiet, rich and full. My angels gathered around me. I saw them, or this time imagined them, smiling like a group of impish school children lined up, posing for a class photograph. I reached into the pocket of my culottes and found one of the special pennies. This time I had put it there myself.

It was a beautifully balanced moment. Nana Bluedress had shown me the way, and I had been able to grow in directions which had made me happier in life than I had ever been.

"Things look good," Bill said.

I got up from my chair with open arms and ran to this wonderful doctor. Tears filling my eyes, I could only say, "Thank you." And in my heart, "Thank you for the breadth of your perspective, your loving manner, and for reconciling the concept of healer with medical doctor."

"School's not out yet," Bill cautioned.

I smiled to myself. "School is never out, I know. I haven't finished with the healing but there is good reason to believe that the load is going to be lighter."

20

With the passage of time I have realized increasingly that it is the healing of a life and a family that is relevant to me. Ambition of all varieties has been a demon for us, manifesting itself in the form of overload, always living the practical, tight life, with little time for savoring life ordinaire, for the expression of love and joy. In daily life we took very little time with one another as a family when it wasn't necessary to do so.

"Cancer is a symbol, as most illness is, of something going wrong in the patient's life, warning him to take another road," Elida Evans' quote reads in Chapter V.

I would modify this to say that there is another approach: with focus and guidance it is possible to seek out and remove serious roadblocks and barriers on a road which might be otherwise perfectly authentic and fine. I feel that it is often the way in which we behave on, use and interpret the road, which needs scrutinizing. Passages need to be cleared for the flow of positive energy removing what Lazaris calls the garbage and the blockages. I have learned that the expression of creativity and love are absolutely crucial in the flow, for example; whereas the dissolution of sorrow (anger and resentment deeply buried) along with fear are the main shibboleths. For me, enthusiasm, fun and adventure are significant positive forces, as well. All of these words are embarrassingly simple to write; they represent a serious, brave challenge, which forms the greater part of the ongoing healing process and fills volumes.

The simile of the three-legged stool is a marvelous one for healing. This is a concept put forth by Dr. Herbert Benson, a Cardiologist affiliated with Harvard Medical School. At one of his healing conferences Dr. Benson explained that healing is like a stool, each leg representing the mind, body or spirit. Each leg needs to be recognized and responsibly addressed for healing to have a chance to be sustained. I see the stool as being constructed of wicker, with legs interwoven, linked to and supporting one another as well as the seat.

In seeking wellness we use the intellect, or mind, most immediately to learn about the disease or situation we are dealing with and to discern which individuals—be they medical practitioners, healers, therapists, family members, or friends—can be most helpful. Perhaps nutritional supplements are a consideration, the foods we choose to eat, or where and how we live. The intellect helps us to become an educated participant in understanding and discerning the best possible choices for healing. Of course the elephant's rope and all that it represents (all of our learned, self-imposed limitations) also lives in the mind, where its role can be revealed and dealt with.

I believe that in terms of disease the body can be a valuable messenger. If the message which the body attempts to deliver goes unnoticed, it has been my experience that the Universe will effectively turn up the volume. "Can you hear it yet? Is this loud (serious) enough for you to respond to?" Once the message is heard the three legs of Dr. Benson's stool come into play.

I also believe that our brains are not the sole receptacles of memory. We park energy in all sorts of places, usually symbolically. Caroline Myss, in her books and tapes, eloquently describes and reaches beyond what many healers have known for a long time. As Lawrence Stoller asked me, years before Carolyn Myss became a known medical intuit and author:

"Do you know what is at the bottom of the illness? Where was the cancer?" Its location was a part of the message.

Energy work is another valuable support for the body, given either by a Reiki practitioner, a hands-on healer, or rolfer, to mention a few. This kind of work helps the healing process by moving old energy out, thereby removing the roadblocks which have collected in our bodies without our realizing it. As someone who works in healing now, I routinely seek this kind of help once a month to clear myself not only of my own negative energy, but of the energy of those I am helping.

The spirit, which I think of as a kind of penumbra of the soul, is for me the strongest, most exciting, and difficult piece. Through the spirit we obliquely express our attitudes and perspectives about the world, and ourselves, the morals and values we live by, and the authenticity of our lives. The will to live is there, as is loving-kindness and connectedness. The spirit wrestles well with the elephant's rope and holds the ultimate truth for the individual, the truth in need of expression. Allowing the spirit to override the intellect drops us into the unknown, where we relinquish control. It is there, often combined with suffering that we have the greatest chance to find wholeness in every way. This is why I always emphasize the value of at least 20 minutes of complete quiet, either in meditation or prayer, each day to give the soul a time in which to speak to us, give us direction, and reconnect us to our lives and our God.

It is not unusual for individuals to circumvent the three-legged challenge, to choose death over facing the pain and fear, perhaps of connubial infidelity, disappointment, or other difficulties in primary relationships. It is dreadful when we find ourselves established in unchosen and disliked professions (perhaps elected to please someone else), or living with a multitude of other points of sorrow or fear. Sometimes, even as people who are seriously ill choose to take on the challenge and live, the disease can be too advanced for the physical life to be saved; but the healing which can occur under these circumstances is often remarkable.

It is important to say that in its unfathomability and vastness, the Divine Mystery can always surprise us. Death, or passing over, as Rosemary Altea would call it, can be something entirely different, bearing little or no relationship at all to what I have described above. An infant dying at birth, a young child dying from leukemia, even a beautiful, fulfilled, connected and giving adult moving on at a young age is often beyond our understanding.

I have an acquaintance in Hong Kong who fairly recently underwent a bout with breast cancer. On a visit there last year we found one another in the old neighborhood supermarket.

"How are you?" I asked with a hug. "You have been in my thoughts. I wondered if you might have returned to Italy. Aren't both of your children in school there now?"

"Yes, they are. But we are staying on. We can't imagine leaving Hong Kong."

"How are you?" I asked again.

"I am fine!" she answered with an almost strident cheerfulness. "I am doing so well. The doctors have encouraged me to get right back into regular life. Being without bosoms is not going to stop me."

I hugged her again.

"Have you thought about changing your life at all?" It was impossible not to ask.

"Definitely not. I like it the way it is."

I smiled, a genuine smile, put my hand on her shoulder and told her how glad I was that she was managing so well, said good-bye, and walked to the check-out counter wondering if I might have said more. Had I acted with loving-kindness? Sometimes it is hard to know.

We all have different timetables, different trains to meet and destinations to reach. In the end there really isn't a right way or a wrong way to do things, just the best way for the individual involved given where they are, where they want to go, and what the Divine Plan has in store for them.

Life now, who we are and who we are becoming seem to me to be key issues in determining the choices we make. That we love God, one another, and ourselves, is the point of being here.

Epilogue

We moved back to America ten years ago. And while I know that all miracles are the same in magnitude and brightness, the miracles that followed were noticeably more obvious and dramatic. They wrapped me up and carried me on ever-deeper into a world imbued with tremendous joy and unvanquished awe. In the backward glance it seems that the experiences put down in *The Elephant's Rope and the Untethered Spirit* were the training wheels for something wider, deeper, larger and more substantial.

The lymphoma reoccurred, but with it ultimate and great treasure. There were extraordinary personal lessons, which accomplished large shifts of consciousness and could fill volumes unto themselves. Having mulled all of this over for some time, I do not believe they could have been accomplished in any other way. Along with grand lessons there were, at times, forthright and simple ones, reinforcing what had been learned so far. There were also the terrifying kick-in-the-backside variety, foundation stones every time. My body suffered and was traumatized but it always bounced back; my spirit claimed its natural place to be.

Our dear friend, Bob Albo, has scratched his head smiling on more than one occasion reflecting on my medical history. To him, the fact that I am still here represents a string of miracles. It goes without saying that he has been an angel in human form, a direct participant. As has wonderful, sagacious Bill Buchholz, beaming over films which showed physical change from time to time as healing work progressed. Bumps disappeared, and a course of chemotherapy combined with a fairly new mono-clonal antibody called Rituxin was significantly shortened because of its mysterious efficaciousness.

Healings of others which I have witnessed and been a part of most recently have been profound. Again, everything deepens, and again there is a surrounding and permeating sense of great blessing and privilege. The choices we make, consciously or unrealized, vibrationally match combined aspects of ourselves at any given point in time. It is both simple and extremely complex. In pragmatic terms everything is vibration. The most important, most powerful of these is love. (Abraham, through Ester Hicks, beautifully describes the power of vibration and the process of harnessing it to our joy and blessing in their extensive body of work. [See Highly Recommended Books.])

This is the place where quantum physics has met the healing world, where what has been called the placebo effect, once correctly understood and supported, will finally receive the honor it deserves. Intention, belief, thought, feelings and emotions are powerful beyond our understanding. It is my belief that as a frontier, this aspect of quantum physics will be more surprisingly significant to mankind, to the planet and to all of life than anything we have discovered or been shown so far.

I have a full healing practice, and with a majority of the proceeds of this book I am in the process of establishing a foundation through which to support my work and the work of others.

I personally work with vibration, with very focused prayer and with subtle organizing energy fields. I have become a Reiki Master, but never taught, and am trained as a Master Dowser. It is part of the Divine plan for all of us to find the tools which suit us best. All we have to do is to want them, to ask for them, and to be open to receive them. After that it is impossible not to use them.

At the moment I am particularly interested in pursuing Gregg Braden's work with the Ancient Essenes (*The Isaiah Effect*, New York: Random House, 2000) in which among other things, Mr. Braden uncovers and explores potency-enhancing aspects of prayer which were omitted when The Bible was compiled in the fourth century a.d.

A short time ago, at the strong suggestion of a friend, I went to see a highly recommended psychic on the Monterey Peninsula, Tricia Emeraude. I hadn't seen anyone since Rosemary Altea in Hong Kong. As it happens, Tricia is also a British lady. "You have such a lot of silver around you," she said at one point in the session. "It is really beautiful."

"I didn't realize," was my answer. "I usually see purple and magenta when I am working."

"Well, I should tell you that there are some rather unhealthy thick silver threads, more like cables, around you which should be cut energetically." She paused. "You must claim more of your life for yourself. The thick threads are supporting people close to you to excess." She closed her eyes. "Heard this before, have you?"

Tricia went quiet. I assumed she was doing some cutting of some kind, but this aspect of energy work is beyond my understanding. I simply sat there thinking about the young woman in Beverly, Massachusetts, who had spoken the same words ten years before. There had been progress, but like so many things, it was like a peeling away of layers. As we think we have taken care of something, it often appears again, perhaps in a watered-down or different version. And sometimes it is the same.

"Watch for the silver, though," Tricia said after a few moments. "You have some work to do in this healing world, and the silver will be a reminder. It is important."

Ultimately, I thanked her and said good-bye.

The very next day, bright and glorious, I was preparing to leave for four days to be with dear friends in Arizona for some much needed healing work and a special study course. Geoff and I took a break and went into town on an errand with our dog.

Then it happened again. I pulled into a parking space, and to the side of the car, as I stepped out, there was something shimmering on the street. Instinctively I stooped down to pick the object up, but didn't know what it was. There was a bizarre, perhaps surreal flash of recognition. It was a penny! But it wasn't. It was silvery. Mr. Lincoln's silhouette was highlighted from behind by copper, but the rest of the coin was definitely silver. Not knowing what to make of it, and being in a bit of a hurry, I actually spoke, "Whatever," and dropped it into a pocket to think about later. It seemed very strange. In the rush I didn't connect the dots. All the same, I put it on my healing altar.

The following afternoon, recanting the most current and perhaps odd episode of the penny story to my healing friends in Flagstaff, Susan Bryant explained it to me.

"It does fit," she said. "It is probably a 1943 penny. There was a shortage of copper during the war, and zinc was used with copper plating," she smiled with one of her broad smiles. "That's what you found." And then she smiled again.

I didn't know about this. My jaw dropped. We were all quiet, and the tears came. Nana Bluedress had outdone herself this time.

All I could say was, "How amazing. How Divine."

It has all been amazing and Divine.

Highly Recommended Books

Abraham-Hicks materials. Abraham-Hicks Publications, P.O. Box 690070, San Antonio, Tex. 78269. Tel: (830) 7552299. Ref. for vibrational work: tapes of 8-28-99 (Kansas City, Mo.), and 9-18-99 (Atlanta, Ga.)

Altea, Rosemary. *The Eagle and the Rose*. (New York: William Morrow & Co., 1996).

_____. *Proud Spirit*. (New York: William Morrow & Co., 1997).

Bailey, Alice. *Esoteric Healing*. (London: Lucis Press Ltd., 1953).

Barnard, Neal, M. D. *Food for Life*. (New York: Crown Trade Paperbacks, 1993).

Braden, Gregg, *The Isaiah Effect*. (New York: Random House, 2000)

Brennan, Barbara. *Light Emerging*. (New York: Bantam Books, 1993).

_____. *Hands of Light*. (New York: Bantam Books, 1998).

Bridge, Ann. *Moments of Knowing*. (New York: McGraw Hill, 1970).

Brodie, Renee. *The Healing Tones of Crystal Bowls*. (Ontario: Aroma Art Ltd., 1996).

Buchholz, William, M.D. *The Medical Uses of Hope,* JAMA, May 2, 1990, Vol. 263, No. 17, p2357-8.

Burnham, Sophy. *A Book of Angels*. (New York: Ballantine Books, 1990).

The Burton Goldberg Group. *Alternative Medicine, The Definitive Guide*. (Washington: Future Medicine Publishing, Inc. 1993).

Buscaglia, Leo. *Living, Loving and Learning*. (New York: Ballantine Books, 1982).

Cameron, Julia. *The Artist's Way*. (New York: G. Putnam's Sons, 1992).

Campbell, Joseph. *The Hero With A Thousand Faces*. (Princeton Univ. Press, 1968).

_____. with Bill Moyers. *The Power of Myth*. (New York: Doubleday, 1998). VIDEO SET is especially valuable.

Canfield, Jack and Mark Hansen. *Chicken Soup for the Soul.* (Florida: Health Communications, 1997).

Chopich, Erika and Margaret Paul. *Healing Your Aloneness: Finding Love and Wholeness Through Your Inner Child.* (New York: Harper & Row, 1990).

Chopra, Deepak, M.D. *Quantum Healing.* (New York: Bantam Books, 1989).

_____. *Magic Body, Magic Mind.* (Illinois: Nightingale-Conant Corp., 1990). AUDIO SET

Course In Miracles, A. (Calif.: Foundation for Inner Peace, 1976).

Cousins, Norman *Anatomy of An Illness.* (New York: W.W. Norton & Co., 1979).

Daniel, Alma and Timothy Wyllie and Andrew Ramer. *Ask Your Angels.* (New York: Ballantine Books, 1992).

deCastillejo, Irene Claremont. *Knowing Woman.* (New York: Harper Colorfon Books, 1973).

Dossey, Larry, M.D *Be Careful What You Pray For.* (San Francisco: Harper San Francisco, 1997).

_____. *Prayer Is Good Medicine.* (San Francisco: Harper San Francisco, 1997).

_____. *Reinventing Medicine.* (San Francisco: Harper San Francisco, 1999).

Duncan, Lois and William Roll, Ph.D. *Psychic Connections.* (New York: Delacorte Press, 1995).

Epstein, Gerals, M.D. *Healing Visualizations: Creating Health Through Imagery.* (New York: Bantam Books, 1989).

Ferguson, Marilyn. *The Aquarian Conspiracy.* (Los Angeles: J.P. Tarcher, Inc., 1980).

Fromm, Erich. *The Art Of Loving.* (New York: Harper and Row, 1956).

Gimbel, Rev. Theo. *Healing With Color and Light.* (Fireside, 1994).

Goodman, Felicitas, Ph.D. *Where the Spirits Ride the Wind.* (Indiana University Press, 1990).

Greene, Brian. *The Elegant Universe.* (New York: W.W. Norton & Co., 1999).

Hay, Louise L. *You Can Heal Your Life.* (Calif.: Hay House, Inc., 1984). AUDIO SET is especially valuable.

Jampolsky, Gerald G., M.D. *Love is Letting Go of Fear.* (New York: Bantam Books, 1970).

_____. *Teach Only Love: The Seven Principles of Attitudinal Healing.* (New York: Bantam Books, 1983).

Kazantzakis, Nikos. *Zorba the Greek.* (London: Faber & Faber Ltd., 1961).

Kornfield, Jack. *A Path With Heart.* (New York: Bantam Books, 1993).

Lawrence, Ron, M.D., Ph.D. and Rosch, Paul J., M.D., *F.A.C.P. Magnet Therapy.* (California: Prima Health, 1998).

Lazaris. *The Sacred Journey: You and Your Higher Self.* (Florida: NPN, 1987).

_____. *Interviews, Book I.* (Beverly Hills: Concept Synergy Publishing, 1988).

_____. *Interviews, Book II.* (Beverly Hills: Concept Synergy Publishing, 1988).

_____. *On Releasing Anger/On Releasing Self Pity and On Releasing Guilt/On Receiving Love.* (Florida: NPN, 1986). AUDIO SET is especially valuable.

LeShan, Lawrence. *You Can Fight For Your Life: Emotional Factors in the Causation of Cancer.* (New York: Evans, 1977).

Levine, Stephen. *Who Dies?* (New York: Anchor Books, 1982).

_____. Healing into Life and Death. (New York: Doubleday, 1987).

Lewis, C. S. *The Four Loves.* (New York: Harcourt Brace Jovanovich, 1960).

Locke, Stephen, M.D., and Douglas Colligan. *The Healer Within.* (New York, Dutton, 1986).

Manning, Matthew. The Link. (Gerrads Cross, [England]: Colin Smythe, Ltd., 1987).

_____. *Guide to Self-Healing.* (London: Thorsons [an imprint of Harper Collins Publishers,] 1989).

_____. *One Foot In The Stars.* (London: Element, 1999).

_____. *Creative Visualization, Just Relax, and The Miracle of Love* are all AUDIO tapes for meditation, available by calling 44-207-938-3788 in England.

Mellody, Pia. *Facing Codependence.* (San Francisco: Harper Collins, 1989).

_____. *The Language of Letting Go.* (San Francisco: Harper Collins, 1990).

Melton, J. Gordon. *New Age Almanac.* (Michigan: Visible Ink Press, 1991).

Miller, Alice. *Thou Shalt Not Be Aware: Psychoanalysis and Society's Betrayal of the Child.* (New York: Farrar, Straus & Giroux, 1984).

_____. *Breaking Down the Wall of Silence.* (New York: Dutton, 1991).

_____. *The Drama of the Gifted Child.* (New York: Basic Books, 1997).

Momaday, N. Scott. *In the Presence of the Sun, Stories and Poems.* (New York: St. Martin's Press, 1992).

Moore, Thomas. *Care of the Soul.* (New York: Harper Collins, 1992).

Myss, Caroline. *Anatomy of the Spirit.* (New York: Random House, 1997). AUDIO TAPE is especially valuable.

Neilhardt, John G. *Black Elk Speaks.* (University of Nebraska Press, 1961).

Newton, Michael, Ph.D. *Journey of Souls.* (Llewellyn Publications, 1998).

Peck, M. Scott, M.D. The Road Less Travelled. (London: Rider, 1983).

_____. *People of the Lie.* (London: Rider, 1985).

Ray, Barbara, Rev. *The Reiki Factor.* (Florida: Radiance Associates, 1983).

Rinpoche, Sigoyal *The Tibetan Book of Living and Dying.* (San Francisco: Harper San Francisco, 1992).

Shine, Betty. *Mind to Mind.* (England: Acacia Press, 1990).

Siebert, Al, Ph.D. *The Survivor Personality.* (New York: The Berkeley Publishing Group, 1996).

Siegel, Bernie, M.D. *Love, Medicine and Miracles.* (New York: Harper & Row, 1989). AUDIO TAPE is especially valuable.

_____. *Peace, Love and Healing.* (New York: Harper & Row, 1989). AUDIO TAPE is especially valuable.

_____. *Prescription for Living.* (New York: Harper Collins, 1998).

_____. Bernie Siegel's web site can be found at www.drbernie.com

_____. *Exceptional Cancer Patients* Org. @ (203) 865-8392.

Simonton, O. Carl, M.D., and Stephanie Matthews-Simonton. *Getting Well Again.* (New York: Bantam Books, 1980). AUDIO TAPE is especially valuable.

Spalding, Baird T. *Life and Teaching of the Masters of the Far East.* (California: De Vorss & Co., 1935).

Wright, Machaelle Small. MAP: *The Co-Creative White Brotherhood Medical Assistance Program.* (Virginia: Perelandra, Ltd., 1990).

Zukav, Gary. *The Seat of the Soul.* (New York: Simon & Schuster, Inc., 1989).